Understanding Dietary Supplements

Understanding Health and Sickness Series
Miriam Bloom, Ph.D.
General Editor

Understanding Dietary Supplements

Jenna Hollenstein, MS, RD, ELS

University Press of Mississippi
Jackson

www.upress.state.ms.us

The University Press of Mississippi is a member of the Association of American University Presses.

First edition 2007

Library of Congress Cataloging-in-Publication Data

Hollenstein, Jenna.
   Understanding dietary supplements / Jenna Hollenstein. — 1st ed.
     p. cm. — (Understanding health and sickness series)
   Includes index.
   ISBN–13: 978–1–57806–980–4 (cloth : alk. paper)
   ISBN–10: 1–57806–980–7 (cloth : alk. paper)
   ISBN–13: 978–1–57806–981–1 (pbk. : alk. paper)
   ISBN–10: 1–57806–981–5 (pbk. : alk. paper) 1. Dietary supplements.
   I. Title.
   RM258.5.H65   2007
   615′.1—dc22   2006035232

British Library Cataloging-in-Publication Data available

Contents

Acknowledgments

I thank Miriam Bloom, Ph.D., editor of the Understanding Health and Sickness Series, for her gentle guidance and persuasive editing, and her daughter, Stephanie Bloom, MD, MPH, for introducing us. Thanks to the reviewers of this book, Jeffrey Blumberg, Ph.D.; Colleen Clemens; Karen Kassel; and Jean Baker, whose comments and suggestions helped bring this book to fruition. Finally, I thank Jeremy, Melissa, Mom, and Dad, for believing all along in my ability to make this book a reality. This book is dedicated to my grandfather, George Hollenstein, who was the first enthusiastic dietary supplement user I knew.

Introduction

Today's educated consumers take an active role in their health. They go to the gym, hire personal trainers, buy and prepare healthful foods, and follow special diets. For many, taking one or more dietary supplements is a natural addition to such healthy behaviors. Some people take dietary supplements casually, while others consider them an integral part of their overall health strategy. The decision to take a dietary supplement may be based on the recommendation of a doctor, dietitian, or friend; a recent television, newspaper, or magazine story; or persuasive marketing materials in the pharmacy or supermarket.

Dietary supplements are often promoted as natural, health-enhancing substances. Many people who take them believe that even if dietary supplements provide no additional health benefit, they can't hurt. Recent findings, however, show that dietary supplements may not be this simple. The common weight-loss dietary supplement ephedra was taken off the market due to serious and sometimes fatal adverse effects; large doses of certain antioxidants were found to have negative effects in specific populations; and, recently, a third large scientific study found that the frequently used herbal cold remedy echinacea had no positive effect on the prevention or severity of colds.

Information regarding dietary supplements abounds. You can find it on the World Wide Web, at specialty stores, at your doctor's or dietitian's office, or at the pharmacy. Even if you don't go looking for it, dietary supplement information may find you, through unsolicited e-mails and pop-up ads; television advertisements and infomercials; and advertising materials in newspapers, magazines, and supermarkets and on other products you normally purchase. The sources of this information are sometimes unclear. Whether from the people selling a product or from scientific experts, information on dietary supplements can be at once persuasive and very confusing. Many consumers are overwhelmed by the information on dietary supplements and need help making sense of it all. Having some background information can make the process of deciding whether to take one or more dietary supplements not only simpler but safer.

Understanding Dietary Supplements is a user's guide. It provides an overall perspective, identifies the important issues, and teaches readers skills to evaluate the growing and ever-changing body of information on dietary supplements. This book is not the definitive text on dietary supplements, nor is it an all-inclusive encyclopedic reference. While such resources can be useful, they quickly become obsolete as new information becomes available. After reading this book, you will be able to make decisions regarding dietary supplements that are relevant to you. Whether you are looking to get started or to organize your thinking about dietary supplements, this book will help you navigate the ocean of dietary supplement information and stay afloat.

In chapter 1, I look at who takes dietary supplements. Surveys have identified trends specific to dietary supplement users, including sex, age, education, geographic region, and health-related beliefs and behaviors. I examine the types of dietary supplements used and the evidence showing whether people who might benefit from dietary supplements are the same people who take them.

In chapter 2, I discuss the regulation of dietary supplements. Dietary supplements are by no means an innovation of the twentieth century, but their regulation is relatively new.

The Dietary Supplement Health and Education Act (DSHEA) administered by the Food and Drug Administration defines dietary supplements and provides a framework for how they should be manufactured, evaluated, marketed, and sold in the United States. I discuss how the Food and Drug Administration manages adverse effects caused by dietary supplements and provide a case study of ephedra, a common weight-loss dietary supplement that was removed from the U.S. market due to serious adverse effects.

In chapter 3, I explore some of the potential safety concerns of taking dietary supplements. As science becomes more sophisticated, the understanding of individual variability has improved. Differences in genetic makeup and consumption patterns (such as diet, drugs, and dietary supplements) among people may influence how dietary supplements act in the body. These differences may also determine whether a dietary supplement provides some benefit, has no positive or negative effect, or causes harm.

In chapter 4, I divide dietary supplements into three groups: vitamin and mineral supplements, herbal and botanical supplements, and other dietary supplements. Although these groups of dietary supplements are all regulated in the same way, they are actually quite different, which can make understanding them extremely complex.

In chapter 5, I provide detailed information about how to evaluate information about dietary supplements. In particular, I describe some general principles for doing research, determining who the experts are, and finding reliable and accurate answers to your questions. Then I provide some final considerations for deciding whether to take one or more dietary supplements and identify those for which there is substantial scientific evidence of a positive effect or no effect.

Material at the end of the book includes a list of current dietary reference intakes for nutrient consumption (Appendix A), an abridged version of the DSHEA (Appendix B), a list of those dietary supplement manufacturers who voluntarily participate in a verification program to ensure the quality and consistency of their products (Appendix C), resources for further research (Appendix D), and a glossary of related terms.

I consulted many resources while writing this book. The Natural Standard (http://www.naturalstandard.com), the Food and Drug Administration (http://www.fda.gov), the Office of Dietary Supplements (http://www.ods.od.nih.gov), and the U.S. Pharmacopeia (http://www.usp.org) were invaluable. Additional resources included *The Honest Herbal: A Sensible Guide to the Use of Herbs and Related Remedies* by Dr. Varro E. Tyler (Pharmaceutical Products Press, 1992), *The Health Professional's Guide to Popular Dietary Supplements* by Allison Sarubin-Fragakis (American Diabetic Association, 2003), and the *Journal of the American Dietetic Association.*

Understanding Dietary Supplements

1. Who Takes Dietary Supplements?

Never before has the United States had a more diverse and bountiful food supply. What food we can't grow or raise, we import—from out-of-season produce to international delicacies. Today, American health professionals seldom puzzle over malnutrition or traditional deficiency disorders brought on by too few nutrients. In fact, too much food is often the problem. Conditions arising from being overweight or obese, such as hypertension, cardiovascular disease, and type 2 diabetes, pose the greatest threat to Americans' health.

The focus of nutrition research, in turn, has shifted to the quality of the diet. Many nutrition scientists are examining how the food we eat affects our health. Some foods, such as those high in saturated and *trans* fats, have negative effects on health, whereas foods such as fruits and vegetables have positive effects. Scientists are also examining individual nutrients and other substances with potential health-promoting properties. Although deficiencies can be avoided by consuming adequate nutrients, it is unclear whether health can be optimized by consuming more than the established adequate nutrient levels.

The idea of "consuming to promote health" has captured many people's imaginations. No longer focusing on eating to prevent nutrient deficiency, American consumers are especially interested in which specific foods, nutrients, and other substances can improve health and quality of life by ameliorating current health conditions or preventing future ones.

Health-seeking individuals purchase food and other items, including dietary supplements, that they believe will make them healthier.

In this chapter, I describe the trends specific to people who take dietary supplements. I extracted data from several sources, including the 2001 and 2005 "Dietary Supplement Barometer Surveys," which were conducted by the Natural Marketing Institute and the Dietary Supplement Education Alliance; the "Nutrition, Health, and Wellness Trends Report," also done by the Natural Marketing Institute; the "Centers for Disease Control and Prevention/National Center for Health Statistics Survey"; the "National Health and Nutrition Examination Surveys"; the *Nutrition Business Journal*; the *Journal of the American Dietetic Association*; and the Council for Responsible Nutrition (http://www.crnusa.org). Most of the figures in this chapter are from the 2001 and 2005 "Dietary Supplement Barometer Surveys." When specific numbers are provided, however, they represent general trends.

Who Takes Dietary Supplements?

The 2005 "Dietary Supplement Barometer Survey" found that 85 percent of Americans regularly took one or more dietary supplements, which represents a sharp increase from the 59 percent reported in the 2001 survey. The *Nutrition Business Journal* estimated that sales of vitamins, minerals, multivitamins, herbal and botanical supplements, sports nutrition supplements, and other dietary supplements totaled $20.3 billion in 2004.

Health-related behaviors are driven by many factors, including sex, age, ethnicity, education, income, geography, and lifestyle, and all of those factors influence the likelihood that an individual will take a dietary supplement. Across

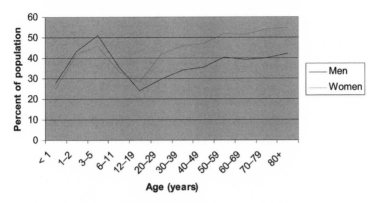

Figure 1.1 Dietary supplement use by age. Adapted from the 2001 "Dietary Supplement Barometer Survey."

nearly all age groups, women are more likely than men to use dietary supplements. In American homes, women still tend to make most of the decisions related to food and nutrition. The nurturing behaviors of women help to explain why they are more likely than men to consume dietary supplements.

Women are also often the main caregivers. Children under 5 years of age, one of the largest age groups to take dietary supplements, tended to get them from their mothers (Fig. 1.1). Evidence suggests that children with special healthcare needs represent a growing population of dietary supplement users. These children are more likely to receive supplements from mothers than from fathers, especially if the mothers are dietary supplement users.

Most people between the ages of 5 and 20 are not consumers of dietary supplements. After age 20, when young adults often begin to take responsibility for their health, more people consume dietary supplements. Women of reproductive age, especially those who are pregnant or planning to become pregnant, are another large group of dietary supplement users.

Table 1.1 Dietary Supplement Use by Education Level

Years of Education	Percent of Population Using Dietary Supplements
0–8	27.8
9–11	31
12	37.8
>12	46.9

Adapted from the 2001 "Dietary Supplement Barometer Survey."

The "National Maternal and Infant Health Survey" found that 81 percent of pregnant women took a multivitamin supplement, most often on the advice of their obstetrician.

After age 20, dietary supplement use increases with age. This is particularly evident among the elderly. More than half of all people over the age of 65 take a multivitamin or other dietary supplement regularly. A substantial proportion of this population also uses herbal supplements regularly. Older Americans who take dietary supplements are already healthier than their counterparts who do not take dietary supplements; they are typically leaner and more physically active, smoke and drink less, and eat more fruits and vegetables.

All surveys indicate that dietary supplement use is highest among non-Hispanic whites, whereas African Americans and Mexican Americans are less likely to consume dietary supplements. Although Asian Americans were not included in the 2005 "Dietary Supplement Barometer Survey," other sources show they are frequent users of dietary supplements. In addition, a language barrier may have prevented surveys from obtaining accurate data from non-English-speaking ethnic groups. In fact, cultural, historic, and anecdotal references suggest that many cultures use nonfood items, including botanical and herbal substances, to treat illness and promote health.

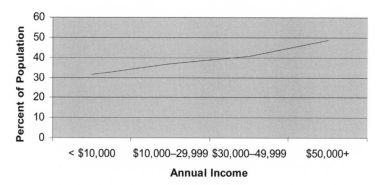

Figure 1.2 Dietary supplement use by income. Adapted from the 2001 "Dietary Supplement Barometer Survey."

People who use dietary supplements tend to be educated and to have a higher than average annual income. Table 1.1 shows a significant difference between dietary supplement use among adults with less than 8 years of education and those with more than 12 years of education. Likewise, there is a direct relationship between annual income and dietary supplement use (Fig. 1.2); a 20 percent increase in dietary supplement use is evident between those whose annual income is less than $10,000 and those who make $50,000 or more annually.

According to the 2001 "Dietary Supplement Barometer Survey," Americans living in the western states have the highest rate of dietary supplement use (47.8 percent). Midwesterners are second (38.0 percent), followed by people living in the Northeast (37.8 percent) and the South (36.2 percent).

Health-Related Behaviors

People who take dietary supplements are likely to be concerned with health-related issues. They eat more fruits and vegetables, exercise more regularly, and smoke and drink alcohol less often than their counterparts who do not take dietary supplements. The 1992 "National Health Interview Survey" found that the diets of dietary supplement users are lower in fat, higher in fiber, and higher in some vitamins and minerals than the diets of nonusers. A 2005 study published in the *Journal of the American Dietetic Association* found that people who take a multivitamin, single-nutrient supplement, and at least one herbal supplement consume more fruits and vegetables than people who only take a multivitamin.

By contrast, a study of people entering the military (mostly young men) showed that the use of ergogenic aids, supplements such as steroid hormones and creatine that are used to increase muscle mass and strength, is associated with high-risk behaviors. People in this group are more likely to drink alcohol and to drink heavily, to ride in a car with a drunk driver or to drive drunk themselves, and to be in a physical altercation.

Across all age groups, most people who take a dietary supplement only consume one product, which is usually a multivitamin. The "National Health and Nutrition Examination Survey III" found that 90 percent of children and 75 percent of teenagers who take dietary supplements only use one product. The 2001 "Dietary Supplement Barometer Survey" showed that about half of people who regularly take dietary supplements take multivitamins (Table 1.2). Another one-third takes single-nutrient dietary supplements, the most popular of which are vitamin C, vitamin E, and calcium. Fewer, but a significant number, take herbal supplements or specialty dietary supplements for specific health or mental health conditions, such as depression. Recent data indicate that use of herbal dietary supplements has reached a plateau or decreased, while the use of condition-specific or specialty dietary supplements has increased.

Table 1.2 Dietary Supplement Use by Type

Supplement	Percent of Supplement Users	Examples
Vitamin/mineral product	46	multivitamin, multivitamin plus minerals, "women's formula" multivitamin
Single-nutrient supplement	35	vitamin C, vitamin E, calcium
Herbal supplement	15	ginseng, garlic, *ginkgo biloba*
Specialty supplement	8	SAM-e (for depression), glucosamine chondroitin (for arthritis)

Adapted from the 2001 "Dietary Supplement Barometer Survey."

Among people with known health conditions, dietary supplement use may differ from that of the general population. A study of more than 600 colon cancer survivors enrolled in a cancer-prevention trial found that 55 percent of them took at least one supplement; among those, 66 percent took more than one product, 13 percent took five or more products, 5 percent took fiber supplements, and about 5 percent took botanical and specialty supplements.

How often users take dietary supplements is somewhat unclear, and estimates vary across surveys. The 1992 "National Health Interview Survey" asked people about daily supplement use, whereas the 1986 survey asked people about dietary supplement use during the prior 2 weeks. The figures from the 1986 survey were substantially larger because they captured both daily and occasional users. The "Slone Survey" found that 40 percent of adults had used vitamin or mineral supplements during the prior week, and a 2001 Council for Responsible Nutrition survey found that 71 percent of people use dietary supplements at least occasionally: 42 percent are regular users, 22 percent are occasional users, and 7 percent are seasonal users.

According to the *Nutrition Business Journal*, while as much as 70 percent of the American population uses supplements, only about 40 percent uses them regularly. About 5 percent of adults are heavy users of dietary supplements, which equates with 10 million people who spend roughly $40 per month; 35 percent are regular users (75 million people who spend about $10 per month); 22 percent are occasional users (50 million people who spend about $4 per month); and 10 percent are rare users (20 million people who spend less than $2 per month on one or two purchases per year).

People are most likely to buy dietary supplements in supermarkets, drug stores, discount department stores, and health food stores (66 percent of total purchases). Others purchase dietary supplements from multilevel marketers (20 percent), through the mail (6 percent) or World Wide Web (2 percent), or from healthcare professionals (6 percent).

Health-Related Beliefs

Whether they are in good health, trying to prevent family medical history from repeating itself, or managing a known illness, people want to feel in control of their health. According to the 2001 "Dietary Supplement Barometer Survey," the top three reasons consumers take dietary supplements are to feel better, prevent sickness, and treat sickness (Table 1.3). Dietary supplement users can be further divided into two groups: those who take them for insurance, which includes people who take dietary supplements for prevention and those who take them to treat an existing condition.

Table 1.3 Reasons for Dietary Supplement Use

Reason	Percent
To feel better	72
To prevent sickness	67
To treat sickness	51
To live longer	50
To build strength and muscle	37
For a specific health reason	36
On the advice of a doctor	30
For sports nutrition	24
To lose or manage weight	12

Adapted from the 2001 "Dietary Supplement Barometer Survey."

Dietary Supplement Use for Prevention

Many people who take dietary supplements are in good health. Sometimes characterized as "the worried well," this population tends to consume healthful diets and dietary supplements and to lead healthy, active lives. While there is no evidence that people in this group rely on dietary supplements as a substitute for good dietary habits, they do believe dietary supplements provide something that may be missing from their diets or that could help them to lead longer, healthier lives.

Among people who use dietary supplements for prevention, some have a more specific agenda. Some take dietary supplements to prevent a specific disease or condition, such as a disease that runs in the family or any disease or condition that has caused the individual concern. If a woman's mother and father died of heart disease, for example, she may use dietary supplements touted to prevent heart disease. However, many health conditions have gained popular attention through the media, and American consumers have responded with heightened awareness. A study by the American Institute for Cancer Research found that 39 percent of people surveyed said they had made changes to their diets to reduce cancer risk, and 68 percent of those reported using dietary supplements. Of the 61 percent of people who had not made changes to their diets, only 36 percent reported using dietary supplements.

Health professionals comprise another large group of dietary supplement users. Doctors, nurses, dietitians, and pharmacists tend to use dietary supplements more frequently than the general public, and they choose dietary supplements according to specific health concerns. One survey of about 4500 female physicians found that half took a multivitamin; those who were at high risk for heart disease were more likely to use antioxidants, and those with a family history of osteoporosis were nearly three times more likely to regularly use a calcium supplement. Among almost 200 cardiologists surveyed in the late 1990s, 44 percent routinely took antioxidants. Within this group, 90 percent took vitamin E, 75 percent took vitamin C, and less than half took beta-carotene. (Unfortunately, this population has not been surveyed since several widely publicized studies linked high intakes of vitamin E and beta-carotene with serious adverse events.)

Dietary Supplement Use for Treatment

The other group of dietary supplement users takes them to treat or manage a current disease. For instance, chondroitin sulfate is used to treat osteoarthritis; saw palmetto is used to treat an enlarged prostate (benign prostatic hypertrophy); and fish oil is used to treat high blood pressure. Despite extensive medical research, many conditions and diseases still have no cure or limited treatment options; other conditions have inadequate treatments and/or treatments that cause adverse effects. Many consumers believe dietary supplements offer an alternative to conventional medicine. Long clinical trials and protracted drug approval processes, which seem to keep valuable information and treatments from people in need, may engender consumer skepticism of traditional medicine, as do fears about drug dependence, adverse effects, and interactions.

Individuals may feel empowered by the choice and ability to take dietary supplements. For them, dietary supplements represent hope when conventional approaches have failed. To be able to take something to promote healthfulness without the written permission of a doctor or pharmacist can provide a sense of autonomy. In addition, dietary supplements have a "natural" connotation, which elicits less fear than a prescription drug synthesized in a factory (although dietary supplements are also manufactured this way).

Consumer Knowledge of Dietary Supplements

Although most consumers believe they have adequate knowledge about dietary supplements, a significant number would like more information about health benefits and think additional information would help them avoid potentially harmful adverse reactions. Other knowledge gaps pertain to specific nutrients, relationships between dietary supplements and disease, and outcomes of taking dietary supplements. In one survey, almost 60 percent of consumers incorrectly answered that it is more important for postmenopausal women to consume the recommended amount of calcium than for people of other ages. (In fact, after age 9, both males and females should consume approximately 1300 mg of calcium daily.) More than 40 percent incorrectly answered that iron supplements provide more energy (only 13 percent of consumers surveyed understood the role of iron, that is, as the oxygen-carrying component of hemoglobin). Twenty-one percent of consumers thought that noticeable effects of dietary supplements can be appreciated after one week, while 12 percent said they did not know how long it would take to see the effects.

According to the 2001 "Dietary Supplement Barometer Survey," 91 percent of consumers said it was important to comply with recommended dosages for prescription drugs, whereas only 71 percent shared this view on dietary supplements. Those surveyed also had surprising opinions about the comparison between dietary supplements and conventional prescription and over-the-counter drugs. About half believed that some supplements are superior to drugs, and about half believed dietary supplements were equivalent to conventional drugs but threatened fewer adverse effects. All of those beliefs are false.

Information from the Natural Marketing Institute showed that more than 70 percent of consumers believed dietary supplements can prevent and treat certain health conditions. While most consumers still choose prescription drugs before dietary supplements to treat a disease or condition, about 40 percent said they would use a combination of prescription drugs, over-the-counter therapies, and dietary supplements as their first choice. About 30 percent of consumers said they would first use only dietary supplements.

A 2002 Harris Poll found that 59 percent thought that dietary supplements must be approved by a government agency before they can be sold to the public. Sixty-eight percent believed that the government required warning labels on supplements with potential adverse effects or dangers, and 55 percent believed that supplement manufacturers cannot make safety claims without solid scientific support. None of these statements is true.

Only half of dietary supplement users tell their doctors about the supplements they are taking. It is unclear whether this is because doctors don't ask or because patients don't tell. What is clear, however, is that this lack of communication prevents doctors and patients from making informed decisions about which dietary supplements, drugs, and behaviors are appropriate and safe.

Do Dietary Supplements Provide a Benefit?

While characteristics such as age and geographic location are related to dietary supplement use, the most striking characteristic about dietary supplement users is that they make health and nutrition a top priority. Therefore, it is important to consider whether people who take dietary supplements benefit from them and whether those people who might benefit from dietary supplements take them.

To consider these questions, I created two diets (Table 1.4) for a hypothetical 50-year-old woman who is 5 feet 6 inches tall, weighs 150 pounds (body mass index of 24.2; a body mass index of 25 is overweight and 30 is obese), is moderately active, and has a daily energy expenditure of approximately 2110 calories. Diets 1 and 2 are similar from the standpoint of total calories, and both diets comprise

Table 1.4 Two Hypothetical Diets for a 50-year-old Woman

Meal	Diet 1	Diet 2
Breakfast	coffee (2 cups each with 1 oz half-and-half and 2 packets sugar) large blueberry muffin (3.5 oz)	multigrain Cheerios (1 cup) low-fat milk (1 cup 1%) raw blueberries (½ cup) orange juice (6 fl oz)
Lunch	6-inch Subway turkey sandwich on white roll mayo (1 Tbsp) regular potato chips (1.0 oz) medium cola (16 fl oz)	lentil soup (10 fl oz) hard-boiled egg (1 large) green salad (1 cup baby spinach leaves, ¼ cup crumbled feta cheese, 1 oz walnuts, and 2 Tbsp olive oil)
Snack	package Peanut M&Ms (1.67 oz)	apple (1 medium) chamomile tea (8 fl oz)
Dinner	rib eye steak (6 oz) medium baked potato (5.5 oz) sour cream (1 oz) iceberg lettuce wedge (1 cup) blue cheese dressing (2 Tbsp) gin martini (4 fl oz)	grilled salmon filet (6 oz) broccoli (½ cup) sautéed in olive oil (1 Tbsp) cooked butternut squash (1 cup) whole wheat pasta (1 cup) red wine (1 glass = 4 fl oz)

one snack and three meals, including dinner at a restaurant. Although I do not recommend evaluating a person's nutrient intake based on one day's diet (and people who occasionally consume poor-quality diets may compensate with variety over time), I am doing this for the purpose of illustration.

Both diets are compared with regard to the percent daily value (%DV) and the tolerable upper limit (UL). The %DV is calculated using the nutrient per serving of food compared with the reference daily intake for that nutrient established by the Food and Drug Administration (FDA; see Table 1.5).

Table 1.5 Comparison of Diets 1 and 2 with Percent Daily Value (%DV) and Tolerable Upper Limits (UL)

Nutrient	Diet 1	%DV	Diet 2	%DV	UL
Calories (Kcal)	2425	121	2203	110	–
Carbohydrate (g)	232.3	77	223.5	75	–
Fiber (g)	9.9	39	28.2	113	–
Fat (g)	104.6	161	101.7	156	–
saturated (g)	34.5	173	21.4	107	–
monounsaturated (g)	27.2	–	45.7	–	–
polyunsaturated (g)	17.9	–	27.8	–	–
Protein (g)	80.3	161	96.2	192	–
Vitamin A (IU)	1125	22	30260	605	9998
Beta-carotene (μg)	208.6	–	12080	–	–
Vitamin C (mg)	40.4	67	186.9	311	2000
Vitamin D (IU)	–	–	164.7	41	50
Vitamin E (mg)	6.6	22	25.2	84	1000
Thiamin (mg)	0.6	37	3.4	226	–
Riboflavin (mg)	1.3	77	3.5	206	–
Niacin (mg)	19.7	99	43.6	218	35
Vitamin B_6 (mg)	1.8	88	4.6	231	100
Folate (μg)	116.1	29	937.8	234	1000
Vitamin B_{12} (μg)	3.2	53	12.7	212	–

(Continued)

Table 1.5 (*Continued*)

Nutrient	Diet 1	%DV	Diet 2	%DV	UL
Vitamin K (μg)	59.6	75	300.8	376	–
Calcium (mg)	228.6	34	929.5	93	2500
Iron (mg)	11	61	30.5	169	45
Magnesium (mg)	177.9	44	509.1	127	350
Potassium (mg)	2524	72	3646	104	–
Sodium (mg)	1904	79	1671	70	–
Zinc (mg)	11.9	79	23.5	156	40
Copper (mg)	0.9	45	1.8	89	10
Selenium (μg)	58	83	108.8	155	400

Kcal, calories; g, gram; IU, International Units; μg, micrograms; mg, milligrams; –, not determined. Diet analysis by www.NutritionData.com. Information is provided only for select nutrients.

The UL is the highest level of a nutrient consumed in one day that is likely to pose no risk of adverse effects. Whether intake of vitamins and minerals above 100 percent of the %DV provides additional benefit is questionable, but exceeding the UL may cause harm. (Appendix A contains a full listing of the updated dietary reference intakes [DRIs]. For more discussion of the DRIs, see chapter 4.) There are no equivalent levels set for other substances such as those found in herbal and botanical dietary supplements. Due to inadequate research and scientific consensus, I cannot comment on their contribution to these diets.

Both diets 1 and 2 meet or exceed established goals for calories, protein, and fat, and both are low in calcium. Diet 1 is low in many nutrients, including fat-soluble vitamins (vitamins A, E, K, and likely D); the B vitamins (thiamine, riboflavin, folate, and vitamins B_6 and B_{12}); several antioxidants (vitamin C and selenium); and minerals (potassium, iron, magnesium, zinc, and copper). A person consuming this diet would therefore be a good candidate for daily supplementation with a multivitamin and/or specialized supplements such as calcium with vitamin D, B-complex vitamins, and antioxidants. However, a person who relies heavily on convenience and prepared foods (as in diet 1) is less oriented to healthful eating and may therefore be less likely to consume these supplements.

Diet 2 exceeds nutrient recommendations for vitamins A, C, and K, the B vitamins, iron, magnesium, zinc, and selenium, and consumption of several nutrients is above the UL. Most worrisome is vitamin A, a fat-soluble vitamin that is stored in the body rather than excreted when consumed in excess, which may be associated with adverse effects. If an individual consuming this diet were to take a dietary supplement (for example, multivitamin or single-nutrient supplements), other nutrient levels could easily exceed potentially harmful levels. A person consuming diet 2, which is composed of whole grains (some fortified), colorful fruits and vegetables, and sources of mono- and polyunsaturated fats (nuts, olive oil, and salmon), makes healthful food choices and is therefore more likely to use dietary supplements.

Many people who take dietary supplements are not lacking nutrients, according to U.S. government recommendations, and little scientific evidence suggests that consuming more than the recommended amounts of some nutrients improves health. Taking dietary supplements to fill a dietary gap, however, is beneficial. Several populations may need dietary supplementation to meet their nutrient goals. The elderly, who require fewer calories as they age, still need to consume high levels of nutrients. One Boston study found that many elderly people did not meet their nutrient needs from diet alone, and a study of the older-old in Georgia found that dietary supplement users and nonusers did not get enough of some nutrients from diet alone. Recent data also suggest that most Americans, especially women and teenage girls, are not consuming adequate amounts of vitamin D.

Experts say a varied, healthful diet is the best way to meet nutritional needs, and consumption of dietary supplements cannot make up for a poor diet. When taken by people who need them, however, dietary supplements can improve nutritional status.

2. The Regulation of Dietary Supplements

One hundred years ago, the dietary supplement industry was very different from today. Production and processing were not standardized, sanitation was questionable (manufacturers had little understanding of bacterial/microbial control and refrigeration was primitive), and distribution was unregulated. The twentieth century brought many changes in how dietary supplements were handled and transported, and several laws sought to improve supplement manufacturing practices.

The U.S. government has long concerned itself with regulation of the substances Americans consume. In the early 1900s, what we now consider to be dietary supplements were regulated as foods. While they are still technically considered foods today, dietary supplements are now regulated by the Dietary Supplement Health and Education Act (DSHEA) under the FDA.

Early Regulation of Dietary Supplements

During the late 1800s and early 1900s, concerns about the safety and purity of the American food supply were mounting. Farmers, millers, trade associations, and drug producers agreed that a government intervention was warranted, but each group was unwilling to compromise its own agenda in the interest of an agreement. In addition to concern about the quality of food that was being sent to American troops fighting in the Spanish-American War, people had qualms about poisonous preservatives and dyes in food and were skeptical about the various health claims for worthless and potentially dangerous patent medicines. Widespread trepidation also came as a result of Upton Sinclair's *The Jungle*, which portrayed the graphic and gory details of Chicago's meat-packing industry.

In 1906 the Pure Food and Drug Act was passed by Congress and signed by President Theodore Roosevelt. The act was created to protect consumers and to provide them with education and choice of products. Essentially, the Pure Food and Drug Act prohibited interstate commerce in misbranded or adulterated foods, beverages, and drugs. Adulteration included removal of valuable components, reduction of overall quality by substituting other ingredients, addition of harmful ingredients, and use of spoiled animal or vegetable products. The act also defined specific labeling requirements; foods and drugs could not be labeled with misleading or false statements, and doing so constituted misbranding. Although the concept of dietary supplements did not yet exist, the Act regulated as foods products that are now known as dietary supplements. Since this first Act, a number of laws have affected the regulation of dietary supplements (Table 2.1).

The 1938 Federal Food, Drug, and Cosmetic Act contained many overriding changes to the 1906 Act, including placing the burden of scientific proof of drug safety and efficacy on the manufacturer, no longer requiring proof of fraud before stopping false claims on drugs, performing food and drug factory inspections, and establishing food standards to "promote honesty and fair dealing in the interest of consumers." During the next several decades, the availability of

Table 2.1 Abridged Timeline of Government Involvement in Food, Drug, and Dietary Supplement Regulation

Year	Legislation or Ruling	Notes
1906	Pure Food and Drug Act	Prohibited interstate commerce in misbranded and adulterated (unwholesome) foods, drinks, and drugs.
1911	United States v. Johnson	The Supreme Court ruled that the 1906 Act did not prohibit false therapeutic claims; it only prohibited false and misleading statements about the ingredients or identity of drugs.
1912	Sherley Amendment	Overturned United States v. Johnson and prohibited labeling medicines with false therapeutic claims intended to defraud the consumer (a step in the right direction, but it created a standard that was extremely difficult to prove).
1914	United States v. Lexington Mill and Elevator Company	The Supreme Court's first ruling on food additives (ban on flour bleached with nitrite residues) placed the burden on the government to prove a food ingredient dangerous.
1938	The Federal Food, Drug, and Cosmetic Act	Extended the government's reach to cosmetics and therapeutic devices; eliminated the Sherley Amendment; required that drugs be demonstrated as safe by the manufacturer prior to marketing; standardized safe tolerances for unavoidable poisons; standardized product identity, quality, and how full a container must be for foods; authorized factory inspections; and introduced court injunctions for violators.

(Continued)

Table 2.1 (*Continued*)

Year	Legislation or Ruling	Notes
1938	Wheeler-Lea Act	The Federal Trade Commission was mandated to oversee advertising for products regulated by the Food and Drug Administration (except for prescription drugs).
1950	Alberty Food Products Co. v. United States	Ruled that directions for use on a drug label must cite the purpose for which the drug is offered, thereby preventing useless and potentially harmful remedies from being marketed without stating purpose.
1958	Food Additives Amendment	Required manufacturers of new food additives to establish and provide data regarding the safety of their products.
1962	Consumer Bill of Rights	John F. Kennedy addressed Congress stating that U.S. citizens were entitled to safety, information, and choice of products, and to be heard regarding their concerns.
1970	Upjohn v. Finch	Determined that commercial success (consumer popularity) of drugs did not constitute evidence of safety and efficacy.
1976	Vitamins and Minerals Amendments	Stopped the Food and Drug Administration from setting standards of potency for vitamins and minerals in food supplements and disallowed regulation of these substances as drugs.

Table 2.1 (*Continued*)

Year	Legislation or Ruling	Notes
1990	Nutrition Labeling and Education Act	Required that all packaged foods bear a standardized label citing ingredients and serving size; also stated that any health claims made on packages must correspond with terms defined by the Secretary of Health and Human Services.
1994	Dietary Supplement Health and Education Act	Defined *dietary supplements* and *dietary ingredients* for the first time, established labeling requirements and a regulatory framework specific to dietary supplements, named the Food and Drug Administration the body that determines good manufacturing practices, and created a commission to recommend how to regulate claims.
2003	Dietary Supplement Current Good manufacturing practices	Good manufacturing practices were proposed for the manufacture and labeling of dietary supplements. (The Food and Drug Administration is still working toward the publication of the current good manufacturing practices final rule.)
2006	Dietary Supplement and Nonprescription Drug Consumer Act	Congress passed a bill that requires manufacturers of dietary supplements and over-the-counter drugs to report all serious adverse effects to the Food and Drug Administration. As of the writing of this book, signature of the bill into law is in the President's hands.

products we now classify as dietary supplements grew exponentially, as did their use.

The Dietary Supplement Health and Education Act

The DSHEA was signed by President Clinton on October 15, 1994. For the first time dietary supplements were given their own set of rules by which to abide. The DSHEA included definitions of *dietary supplement* and *new dietary ingredient* and provided for the creation of a commission to advise on the regulation of these substances.

Important Definitions

According to the DSHEA, a *dietary supplement* is a product that

- is intended to supplement the diet;
- contains one or more dietary ingredients (including vitamins, minerals, herbs or other botanicals, amino acids, and other substances) or their constituents;
- is intended to be taken by mouth as a pill, capsule, tablet, or liquid;
- is not represented as a conventional food or as a food replacement;
- is labeled on the container's front panel as being a dietary supplement;
- includes products such as an approved new drug, certified antibiotic, or licensed biologic that was marketed

as a dietary supplement or food before approval, certification, or license (unless waived by the secretary of the Department of Health and Human Services).

The DSHEA presumes that ingredients introduced prior to October 15, 1994, are safe. A *new dietary ingredient*, on the other hand, is an ingredient not sold in the United States in a dietary supplement prior to that date or one that is part of a dietary supplement introduced on or after October 15, 1994. At least 75 days before marketing a dietary supplement containing a new dietary ingredient, manufacturers must provide the FDA with their basis for deeming the ingredient "reasonably expected to be safe."

If they meet the criteria above, botanicals may be considered dietary supplements. A *botanical* is a plant, or part of a plant, that is used for one or more of its specific characteristics, including medicinal properties, flavor, and scent; *herbs* are a subset of this group, usually the green, leafy portion of the plant. Botanicals are identified by Latin names designating the genus and species of the plant. Many botanicals, however, have numerous common names or are identified only by their genus. For example, the commonly known dietary supplement black cohosh (*Cimicifuga racemosa*) is also known as baneberry, black snakeroot, bugwort, cohosh bugbane, rich weed, rattle root, solvlys, and squaw root, to name a few. Botanicals can be sold in many forms, including fresh or dried, as liquid or solid extracts, in tablets and capsules, as loose powders, and in tea bags. Table 2.2 describes common preparations of botanicals.

The intended use of a consumable product is essentially what determines its classification—and therefore its regulation—as a food, drug, or dietary supplement. Drugs are created to treat, cure, or somehow mitigate a disease or

Table 2.2 Common Preparations of Botanicals

Preparation	Process	Product
Tea	Also known as an infusion, a tea is made by adding boiling water to fresh or dried botanicals and steeping them.	a liquid that can be drunk hot or cold
Decoction	Sometimes botanicals are more aggressively processed. A decoction is made by simmering botanicals in boiling water for longer periods of time.	a liquid that can be drunk hot or cold
Tincture	A botanical is soaked in a solution of alcohol and water to make a tincture. Tinctures both concentrate and preserve botanical substances, and they can be identified by the concentration of botanical substance in the final product.	a liquid that can be drunk (diluted or as a concentrate)
Extract	A botanical is soaked in a liquid to extract certain chemicals and the extract is concentrated.	can be consumed as a liquid, in capsules, or as tablets containing the evaporated substance

condition. A dietary supplement cannot claim to have these effects; if such a claim is made by the manufacturer of a dietary supplement, the substance must then be regulated as a drug. However, a manufacturer can claim a supplement is "used for" anything at all, even though it may have no effect.

Labeling

Labels must include the word *supplement* and identify the product as a dietary supplement. The required information on

Supplement Facts

Serving Size 1 tablet
Servings Per Container 250

Amount Per Serving	%Daily Value*
Calcium (as dicalcium phosphate) 68 mg	7
Ginkgo biloba Leaf Extract 60 mg (Standardized to 24% Ginkgo Flavonglycosides & 6% Terpenelactones)	**

* Percent Daily Values are based on a 2000 calorie diet.
** Daily Value not established

OTHER INGREDIENTS: Microcrystalline
Cellulose, Glyceryl Monostearate,
Magnesium Stearate.

Figure 2.1 *Ginkgo biloba* dietary supplement label

dietary supplement labels includes the name and quantity of each nutrient and dietary ingredient or, for proprietary blends, the total quantity of all dietary ingredients (except inert ingredients) in the blend. Since 1997 all supplements must bear a label entitled "Supplement Facts," which is very similar in format and content to the "Nutrition Facts" label that appears on all food and beverages marketed in the United States. Labels on herbal and botanical products must state which part of the plant the contents come from. Figure 2.1 shows a sample label from a bottle of *Ginkgo biloba*.

Some dietary supplements are included in official compendia, such as the U.S. Pharmacopoeia, the Homeopathic Pharmacopoeia of the United States, or the National Formulary. If a supplement is included in a compendium, it must correspond with the specifications of that compendium. For dietary supplements not included in official compendia, the label must correctly identify each substance and the amount in the supplement.

Dietary supplement labels must also contain nutritional information, including ingredients present in significant amounts, and first listing those for which the FDA has established %DVs. Labels must also include the quantity per serving for each dietary ingredient and may include the source of the ingredients.

The FDA published the *Dietary Supplement Labeling Guide* in 2005. This guide was created in response to numerous questions from the dietary supplement industry regarding all legislation relevant to dietary supplement labels.

Health Claims on Dietary Supplement Labels

The use of health claims on food products is regulated by the Nutrition Labeling Education Act of 1990 (see Table 2.1). Health claims describe the relationship between a specific nutrient and a disease or condition. In order to appear on the food or dietary supplement label, health claims must be evaluated and preapproved by the FDA based on "significant scientific agreement." Few such health claims have been authorized by the FDA.

While a dietary supplement can never be claimed to "diagnose, prevent, mitigate, treat, or cure" a specific disease, the DSHEA allows use of specified statements on the labels of dietary supplements. In addition to the approved health claims listed in Table 2.3, dietary supplement labels can contain statements about nutritional support. These statements, known as *structure-function claims*, may describe how the product affects the structure or function of the body or the overall well-being of the consumer (Table 2.4). Before making such statements on a label, however, manufacturers of dietary supplements must prove that the nutritional support statement is truthful and not misleading, and they

Table 2.3 Food and Drug Administration-Authorized Health Claims

Diet/Disease Claim	Approved Claim	Dietary Supplements Permitted to Display Claim
Calcium and osteoporosis	Regular exercise and a healthy diet with enough calcium help teen and young adult white and Asian women maintain good bone health and may reduce their risk of osteoporosis.	some calcium supplements
Folate and neural tube defects	Healthful diets with adequate folate may reduce a woman's risk of having a child with a brain or spinal cord birth defect.	some dietary supplements containing folate
Dietary soluble fiber and coronary heart disease	Diets low in saturated fat and cholesterol that include 3 grams of soluble fiber from whole oats per day may reduce the risk of heart disease.	dietary supplements containing psyllium seed husk
Plant stanol and plant sterol esters and coronary heart disease	Diets low in saturated fat and cholesterol that include two servings of foods that provide a daily total of at least 3.4 grams of plant stanol esters in two meals may reduce the risk of heart disease.	dietary supplements in soft gel form

These claims are current as of the writing of this book.

must notify the FDA within 30 days of making the statement. When a nutritional support statement appears, the label must also state, "This statement has not been evaluated by the Food and Drug Administration. This

Table 2.4 Examples of Allowed Structure/Function Claims on Dietary Supplements

Structure/Function Claim	Dietary Supplement
Promotes healthy gums, capillaries, and teeth	vitamin C tablets
Supports healthy liver function and detoxification	super milk thistle caplets
Supports the immune system	vitamin C chewable tablets

product is not intended to diagnose, treat, cure, or prevent any disease."

Additional Information Given to Consumers

Manufacturers of dietary supplements often seek to promote their product by providing supporting material such as a scientific study or the statement of a medical or nutrition professional. Under certain conditions, this additional material is not considered to be "labeling," per se, and is therefore not regulated in the same fashion.

If the manufacturer uses a reprinted scientific article, it must be printed in its entirety and must not be accompanied by any added information. Additional publications used in connection with the sale of dietary supplements cannot be misleading, cannot promote a particular manufacturer or brand, must present a balanced view of the available scientific evidence, and must be physically separate from the dietary supplements in the store.

Good Manufacturing Practices

The DSHEA gave the FDA the authority to establish special good manufacturing practices for dietary supplements. In

March 2003 the FDA released its "Proposed Rule for Dietary Supplement Current Good Manufacturing Practices," which addresses important components of dietary supplement manufacture, including design and construction of manufacturing facilities, quality-control procedures, testing of the final product(s) or incoming and in-process materials, management of consumer complaints, and record keeping and filing of compliance with these standards. The basic tenets of the current good manufacturing practices require that dietary supplement manufacturers use current industry standards in the processing of dietary supplements to avoid contamination (by pesticides, heavy metals, or other impurities) and improper labeling and to ensure that product labels accurately reflect the identity, purity, quality, strength, and composition of dietary supplements. The following are some examples of product quality problems that these rules are meant to address:

- contains more of the active or inactive ingredients than listed on the label;
- contains less active ingredients than listed on the label;
- contains the wrong ingredient(s);
- contains a drug contaminant;
- contains other contaminant(s), such as bacteria, mold, pesticide, or lead;
- package contains foreign material, such as glass;
- improper packaging and/or mislabeled product.

The "Proposed Rule for Dietary Supplement Current Good Manufacturing Practices" was open to public comment for a year before it was to be considered final. After approval, dietary supplement companies would have 36 months to implement the changes necessary to comply with the rule. Until then, dietary supplement manufacturers were to follow good manufacturing practices for foods. During the comment period, however, the FDA received more than 1600 pages from consumers and members of the dietary supplement industry. A final rule therefore has been delayed and is expected in late 2006 (for current information, see http://www.cfsan.fda.gov/~dms/ds-ind.html#GMPS).

Creation of New Government Entities

Appointed in 1995, the Commission on Dietary Supplements directs the labeling of dietary supplements, essentially to determine how to provide scientifically valid information about them. The first commission comprised scientists from various U.S. universities with expertise in dietary supplements, a member of the Council for Responsible Nutrition, a Seton Hall University School of Law professor, a public relations specialist, and a representative from the Herb Research Foundation.

Responsibilities carried out by the Commission on Dietary Supplements are now being performed by the Office of Nutritional Products, Labeling, and Dietary Supplements' Division of Dietary Supplement Programs, which comprises a regulations and review team, a compliance and enforcement team, and a clinical review team. Led by Dr. Susan Walker, the division creates policies, regulations, and guidance documents to ensure the safe manufacture and labeling of dietary supplements and reviews safety information submitted by dietary supplement manufacturers 75 days before the marketing of a product to ensure that it is reasonably expected to be safe.

The DSHEA also called for the creation of the Office of Dietary Supplements (ODS), which is housed within the National Institutes of Health and is responsible for facilitating research into the role of dietary supplements in disease prevention and health promotion. The mission of ODS is to strengthen knowledge about dietary supplements by evaluating available research and stimulating and supporting more scientific trials, as well as by educating people about the current state of knowledge. As part of their mission, ODS hosted the 2000 National Nutrition Summit and created numerous resources, including Computer Access to Research on Dietary Supplements, International Bibliographic Information on Dietary Supplements, Annual Bibliographies of Significant Advances in Dietary Supplement Research, and Dietary Supplement Ingredient and Labeling databases (see Appendix D). The ODS's 2004–2009 strategic plan comprises five major goals: (1) expanding the evaluation of dietary supplements in reducing the risk for chronic disease; (2) fostering research on dietary supplements for optimal health and performance; (3) enhancing understanding of the basic effects of dietary supplements on biological systems; (4) improving methodologies; and (5) expanding outreach and education.

Adverse Effects of Dietary Supplements

The FDA has the burden of proving that a dietary supplement is adulterated, that it "presents a significant or unreasonable risk of illness or injury." The FDA, however, must rely on the honesty of the industry to ensure safety. Through scientific studies, dietary supplement manufacturers determine that their ingredients present no significant or unreasonable risk to consumers and submit that information to the FDA. Although the FDA does not participate in or oversee the testing of dietary supplements for safety, the FDA is responsible for removing unsafe dietary supplements from the market.

Adverse or suspected adverse effects of dietary supplements should be reported to the FDA. Once the FDA receives such information, it generates alerts and warnings for consumers and letters notifying the manufacturer that their dietary supplement may be associated with harmful adverse events. The results of these actions may range from a consumer warning, labeling change, or product recall to a full-fledged product withdrawal. Dietary supplement manufacturers may voluntarily recall a product, as in the case of a labeling error, product mix-up, contamination, or questionable stability of the product or its components. The FDA may also request or order a product recall based on the above criteria.

Product recalls are expensive and done because there is something wrong with the product. The type of recall for dietary supplements depends on the severity of potential adverse effects. A class I recall means there is reasonable evidence to suggest that use of a product will cause serious adverse effects or death; a class II recall means a product may cause temporary or treatable adverse effects or that the risk of serious adverse effects is low; and a class III recall means the adverse effects are not likely to be serious.

Below is an adaptation of a letter from the FDA's Office of Nutritional Products, Labeling, and Dietary Supplements to the distributor of a hazardous dietary supplement.

Dear Mr. Doe,

Your product, *Dietary Supplement X (DSX),* has been implicated in a number of serious adverse reactions, specifically serious liver injuries. Our evaluation of the complaints of serious injuries associated with the use of *DSX* shows that it is associated with acute hepatitis when used under the conditions of use recommended on the label. The FDA has received multiple reports of persons who developed acute hepatitis and/or liver failure with the use of *DSX*.

Given the serious hazard presented by the use of your product, we strongly recommend that you take prompt action to remove *DSX* from the market. Further, the FDA urges you to alert your customers to immediately stop using *DSX*. Toward this end, the FDA has issued a consumer warning to alert consumers to the serious risks presented by the use of your product, *DSX*.

Should you have any questions or require any FDA assistance, contact Dr. John Smith of my staff.

The response of the dietary supplement manufacturer to such notification varies. Ideally, the manufacturer would remove its product from the market and warn consumers about potential dangers through its web site and at places where the product was sold. This process could take months or even years, however, posing the risk of additional adverse events. The FDA is mandated to intervene only when adverse effects are numerous and severe and the dietary supplement manufacturer continues to make the product available to consumers despite FDA warnings. The following case study reviews events resulting in the removal of dietary supplements containing ephedra from the U.S. market.

The Ephedra Recall

In *The Honest Herbal*, Dr. Varro E. Tyler wrote that ephedra (*Ephedra sinica*) might have been the first Chinese herbal remedy to have been used significantly in western medicine. A potent central nervous system stimulator, ephedra (also known as *ma huang*) is effective as a nasal decongestant and can provide relief of congestion and bronchiole constriction to people suffering from asthma. The man-made equivalents of ephedra, ephedrine and pseudoephedrine, have been added to many over-the-counter cold and asthma medications. *Ephedra sinica* stimulates the heart and causes constriction of the blood vessels, which raises blood pressure.

Ephedra began to be used as a weight-loss aid in the mid-1970s. This may have been the result of recommendations by natural health practitioners and/or the observation that ephedra had a "speed-like" effect on the body, which people might have interpreted as an ability to increase metabolism. Dietary supplements with ephedra often contained additional stimulants such as caffeine. Those products were marketed as weight-loss supplements that conveyed an "energy boost." In the 1990s, the dietary supplement industry estimated that as many as 3 billion servings of dietary supplements containing ephedra were being consumed each year in the United States.

Gradually, dietary supplement manufacturers and the FDA received numerous reports of adverse effects from consuming ephedra. Serious adverse effects of ephedra use include rapid heart rate, high blood pressure, arteriole constriction, seizure, stroke, and sudden death. In 1996 the FDA released a statement that consumers should avoid ephedra-containing dietary supplements. At that time, more than 800 deaths in the United States were attributed to their use.

In 1997 the FDA proposed revisions that would require all ephedra-containing products to be labeled with the following: "taking more than the recommended serving may result in heart attacks, seizures, or death." The FDA also proposed that all products be limited to 8 mg of active ingredient per serving, with a maximum daily dose of 24 mg; use should not exceed 7 days; and consumers should not use the supplement in combination with other specified substances that exacerbate the effects, such as caffeine. In the summer of 1999, however, the U.S. General Accounting Office reported that, although the FDA was justified in voicing concerns over the safety of dietary supplements containing ephedra, more evidence was needed before regulations could limit dosage and duration of use. Several months later, despite 140 additional deaths attributed to ephedra, the FDA capitulated.

In response to growing concern among consumers and government entities, members of the Ephedra Committee of the American Herbal Products Association launched a public relations group called the Ephedra Education Council. In 2002 the council released a report of fifty-five clinical studies citing beneficial effects of ephedra when taken as directed, with zero studies showing evidence of adverse effects.

By 2003 additional studies had noted the risks of ephedra, including a report by the Rand Corporation, which conceded sufficient cause for concern regarding the relationship between consumption of ephedra and adverse events, including nausea, vomiting, heart palpitations, and psychiatric symptoms (anxiety and mood changes). When Steve Bechler, a 23-year-old pitcher for the Baltimore Orioles, died from an ephedra-related adverse event in February 2003, the national media began to report the risks of ephedra consumption.

Illinois banned the sale of products containing ephedra in 2003. Several other states considered similar legislation, restricted the sale to those over 18 years of age, or required products to have warning labels. Several sports organizations banned the use of dietary supplements containing ephedra, and General Nutrition Centers, the largest national dietary supplement store, discontinued the sale of products containing ephedra.

On February 6, 2004, the FDA issued a final rule that prohibited the sale of dietary supplements containing ephedra (ephedrine alkaloids) because they presented a significant and unreasonable risk of illness or injury. This rule became effective 60 days after the date of publication. Since then, individual manufacturers of dietary supplements containing ephedra have challenged the FDA's ruling, and the FDA has developed analytical methods by which they can determine whether a dietary supplement contains ephedra. Dietary samples that test positive for ephedra undergo additional analysis to confirm those results.

In April 2005 a federal district court in Utah struck down the ban on the sale of ephedra, citing inconclusive evidence that it is harmful at lower doses (and therefore that the FDA lacked the authority to effect such a ban). While dietary supplement manufacturers were legally permitted to sell products containing ephedra (within certain limitations of potency and labeling), the company responsible for initiating this appeal elected to not reintroduce these products into the market. The FDA appealed this ruling, and a U.S. court of appeals ruled in their favor on August 17, 2006. However, ephedra-containing dietary supplements can still be purchased, mostly from Internet distributors.

While the FDA works to ensure that dietary supplement manufacturers adhere to the DSHEA, the volume of dietary supplements available makes this surveillance extremely difficult. In addition, the magnitude of evidence necessary for the FDA to effect any action against manufacturers of potentially harmful dietary supplements is so great, many people view the DSHEA as ineffective and, in fact, a deregulation.

3. The Safety of Dietary Supplements

Dietary supplement safety should be of primary concern to consumers. Because they are assumed to be safe unless proven otherwise, dietary supplements present special safety challenges. In 2000 the FDA received 500 dietary supplement adverse event reports; that number rose to 553 in 2001 and to 1214 in 2002. Adverse events caused by dietary supplements vary from mild to severe and may be influenced by individual health status (medical history and genetic makeup), dietary supplement composition and dosage (including levels of active and inactive ingredients), and concomitant consumption of other substances (including foods, beverages, over-the-counter and prescription drugs, and other dietary supplements).

Health Status

Dietary supplements may act differently in different people. As noted by Christine Lewis-Taylor, former director of the FDA's Office of Nutritional Products, Labeling, and Dietary Supplements, "one man's dose can be another man's poison." An individual's genes and health status help to explain this difference.

Nutritional genomics and metabalomics are growing areas of research that explain the relationship between genetic makeup and nutrition- and metabolism-related outcomes.

Certain relationships between nutrients and health outcomes are well characterized. Folate supplementation, for example, is recommended for all women of childbearing age to prevent fetal neural tube defects. By isolating and analyzing the function of the genes responsible for folate metabolism, however, scientists have identified a genetic variation that predisposes some women to give birth to babies with neural tube defects. This knowledge may eventually allow scientists to target folate supplementation to at-risk individuals.

Stage of life, medical history, and environmental factors such as diet and exercise can affect how a dietary supplement behaves in the body. Several populations are at increased risk of adverse effects of dietary supplements:

- children,
- people of smaller stature,
- elderly people,
- women who are pregnant or breastfeeding,
- people with immune disorders (for example, HIV or AIDS),
- people with cancer,
- malnourished people,
- people with existing or subclinical liver or kidney disease,
- people with a history of gastrointestinal health conditions (such as Crohn's disease) or surgery (such as gastric bypass surgery),
- people who are hospitalized,
- transplant recipients,
- surgical patients.

While research has revealed the unique nutritional needs in women of childbearing age (for example, 400 micrograms of folate are recommended to prevent neural tube defects in offspring, and if pregnant, supplemental vitamins are recommended), information on the effects of dietary supplements during pregnancy and breastfeeding are extremely limited. This is largely due to ethical considerations: scientific studies are not conducted during pregnancy and breastfeeding because of potential risks to the women and their babies. Several herbal dietary supplements historically used during pregnancy have been identified as harmful (Table 3.1).

Certain dietary supplements may cause adverse effects during surgery, including increased or decreased bleeding (Table 3.2). Medical or surgical professionals should be consulted several weeks before any scheduled surgery to determine whether dietary supplements should be discontinued.

Perhaps the most common adverse effects of dietary supplements are gastrointestinal, including constipation, diarrhea, or nausea. Gastrointestinal adverse effects are often present when a dietary supplement is first added to the diet. Over time, these symptoms may decrease or may cause an individual to discontinue use.

Table 3.1 Potential Adverse Events Associated with Some Herbal Dietary Supplements during Pregnancy

Herbal Dietary Supplement	Potential Outcome
Ginger (in amounts greater than those found in food, >1 g dry)	abortion, birth defects, increased bleeding
Blue cohosh tea	fetal heart attack
Birthwort	kidney toxicity
Hellebore, hemlock, or tragacanth	birth defects (demonstrated in animals)

Table 3.2 Dietary Supplements That May Alter Bleeding

Increased Bleeding	Decreased Bleeding (Increased Clotting)
Black cohosh	Coenzyme Q10
Chondroitin sulfate	Melatonin
Dong quai	Vitamin K
Fish oil	
Garlic	
Ginger	
Ginkgo	
Saw palmetto	
St. John's wort	
Vitamin E	

Note: This table is not all-inclusive.

Many dietary supplements are metabolized by the liver and/or kidneys and may therefore cause adverse effects in people with overt or subclinical liver or kidney disease. Adverse effects could include worsening of disease complications or presentation of a previously undiagnosed disease. Other dietary supplements may cause adverse effects in other parts of the body; for example, calendula may cause eye irritation, *Ginkgo biloba* can cause skin to become dry, and St. John's wort may increase sensitivity to the sun. Table 3.3 lists several potential adverse effects caused by dietary supplements.

Dietary Supplement Composition

Variability

Dietary supplements are natural substances that may contain variable amounts of active and inactive ingredients. These amounts depend on several factors, including the age and

Table 3.3 Types of Adverse Events

Body System	Symptoms
Cardiovascular	increased/decreased heart rate, increased/decreased blood pressure, palpitations, arrhythmia, heart attack, transient ischemic attack (TIA), stroke, sudden death
Dermatologic	dermatitis/rash, dryness, photosensitivity, changes in nails
Endocrine	hyperglycemia, hypoglycemia, changes in lipid levels, hypothyroidism, changes in insulin levels, changes in sex hormone levels
Gastrointestinal	diarrhea, constipation, cramping, belching, bloating, nausea, vomiting, heartburn, anorexia, bowel obstruction
Genitourinary	decreased fertility, increased urinary urge
Hematologic	thrombocytopenia, increased bleeding risk, increased clotting risk, altered blood chemistry
Hepatic	hepatitis, hepatotoxicity
Neurological	seizure, sedation, central nervous system depression, dizziness, headache, diaphoresis, fever/chills
Ocular	dryness, irritation, blurred vision, conjunctivitis, cataract
Renal	kidney stones, nephritis, nephropathy, protein in the urine, kidney failure
Respiratory	exacerbation of asthma, shortness of breath
Skeletal/muscular	changes in bone mineral content, muscle weakness

Note: This table is not all-inclusive.

specific part of the plant, the composition of the soil in which it was grown, the time of year it was harvested, and how the substance was processed and stored. While manufacturers must label their products with the contents, the recommended daily dose, and how much of the active ingredient each dose contains, dietary supplement composition can vary widely. From bottle to bottle, batch to batch, year to year, and company to company, consumers may not be aware of exactly what they are consuming.

In a 2003 study published in *Archives of Internal Medicine*, researchers analyzed 880 herbal dietary supplements collected from a variety of sources, including grocery stores, retail pharmacies, discount stores, and health food stores. They compared the dietary supplement ingredients and the recommended daily doses stated on the label with their own laboratory analyses. Of the products sampled, 43 percent were consistent with a standardized pharmacy reference for ingredients and recommended daily doses, 20 percent were consistent regarding ingredients only, and 37 percent were either inconsistent or did not contain enough information on the label to determine consistency. The authors suggested that much of this inconsistency could be attributed to insufficient research on the part of the manufacturer and inadequate understanding of how to ensure consistency in a natural resource.

A study presented at the Sixth International Cartilage Repair Society Symposium in 2006 analyzed ten commercially available dietary supplements containing chondroitin sulfate, which is commonly used to improve joint pain associated with osteoarthritis. Researchers evaluated the ability of the raw materials to inhibit gene expression of three substances involved in cartilage breakdown. These results were compared with a reference standard, which was the chondroitin sulfate supplement used in a previous study, the largest federally funded trial evaluating the supplement's clinical effects. Only one of the ten supplements inhibited gene expression in a manner equivalent to the reference standard. Two of the supplements had no detectable effect, and the remainder had inconsistent effects on gene expression.

Contamination

Dietary supplements may contain harmful or undesirable substances such as pesticides or heavy metals. Contaminants may be present before a substance is harvested for use as a dietary supplement or may be introduced during processing and packaging.

For example, coral calcium, a dietary supplement said to contain remnants of living coral reefs, may contain significant and harmful amounts of lead and other heavy metals. Consumption of excessive levels of lead can cause neurological problems, increased blood pressure, reproductive impairment, and hearing and sight problems. Scientists are also concerned that people who are allergic to shellfish may experience serious adverse events such as hives, swelling, and breathing problems, because of the presence of these allergens in coral reefs.

In 2003 the Sports Nutrition Working Group of the International Olympic Committee Medical Commission reported that approximately one in five dietary supplements commonly used by athletes were contaminated. Protein powders; amino acid supplements; creatine; pyruvate; and several vitamin, mineral, and herbal supplements were found to contain steroid-like chemicals that were not identified on product labels, caused positive doping tests, and were not known to be safe.

Dietary supplements may also contain controlled substances. Acetaminophen, aspirin, antihistamines, and corticosteroids have been found in dietary supplements that did not list them as ingredients. In 2005 the FDA issued a warning about a dietary supplement that contains the antidiabetic agent glyburide after it caused hypoglycemia (dangerously low blood sugar) in several consumers. In 2006 the FDA warned consumers against using several weight-loss dietary supplements that contain chlordiazepoxide HCl (the active ingredient in the drug Librium) and fluoxetine HCl (the active ingredient in the antidepressant Prozac).

Dietary Supplement Interactions

A 1997 survey published in the *Archives of Internal Medicine* indicated that 18 percent of prescription drug users were also using herbal or vitamin and mineral dietary supplements. The authors estimated that this placed approximately 15 million people at risk of interactions between drugs and dietary supplements, 3 million of whom were 65 years and older.

The results of a 2005 survey published in the *Journal of the American Dietetic Association* indicated that as the use of non-vitamin, non-mineral supplements (such as herbal and botanical dietary supplements) had increased during the previous 10 years, so had the concomitant use of dietary supplements and over-the-counter and/or prescription drugs. Many of the people who participated in the survey were taking multivitamin pills and were surprised to learn that their multivitamins contained non-vitamin, non-mineral dietary (that is, herbal and other) supplements as well.

Interactions with Drugs

Few studies have specifically examined interactions between drugs and dietary supplements in the general population, and existing reports have found only mild interactions. These articles comprised mainly case reports, estimations based on laboratory experiments (not in humans), and speculation based on pharmacology studies and theoretical risks. Lack of data, however, does not imply lack of danger.

Dietary supplements may alter the activity of conventional drugs. Such interactions may occur in individuals who are particularly sensitive or immunocompromised or for drugs that have a narrow therapeutic window. In addition, response to drug and dietary supplement consumption may change with age and health status. Interactions between drugs and dietary supplements are especially likely in geriatric patients because they use more drugs and often combine prescription and over-the-counter drugs with herbal remedies. People with a chronic illness, specifically those with hepatic or renal impairment, are at higher risk of harmful interactions between drugs and dietary supplements.

Drug concentration or activity in the blood may be increased if a dietary supplement aids the absorption of the drug or if it inhibits enzyme destruction or elimination of the drug. Conversely, drug concentration and/or activity in the blood may be decreased if the dietary supplement binds components of the drug, thus preventing its absorption, or if the dietary supplement stimulates production and/or activity of enzymes that destroy the drug.

Some of the most popular dietary supplements may interact with drugs. A 2004 study at the University of Chicago Medical Center, which was funded by the National Institutes of Health and the Tang Center for Herbal Medicine Research, found that ginseng, which is commonly taken to enhance well-being, reduce fatigue, and improve immune response, decreased the effect of the anticoagulant warfarin. People who consumed warfarin and ginseng had an increased incidence of blood clots and therefore an increased risk of deep vein thrombosis. Because of ethical reasons, this study was done in healthy individuals, but the researchers believed that the results could be applied to those taking warfarin for prevention of deep vein thrombosis.

St. John's wort, which people commonly take for mild to moderate depression, may alter the effectiveness of drugs prescribed for HIV, heart disease, depression, epileptic seizures, and cancer and may interfere with oral contraceptives. Dietary supplements containing garlic have the potential to increase the risk of bleeding if combined with other drugs that increase bleeding risk, such as aspirin and warfarin. Specific interactions are listed in Table 3.4, but additional resources should be consulted to determine your risk of drug–dietary supplement interactions (see Appendix D).

Table 3.4 Dietary Supplements and Potential Interactions

Dietary Supplement	Interaction(s)
Black cohosh	antihypertensive drugs: may further reduce blood pressure anticoagulants: may increase bleeding risk
Chondroitin sulfate	anticoagulants: additive effects may increase risk of bleeding
Coenzyme Q10	antihypertensives: additive effects may further lower blood pressure anticoagulants: antagonistic effects may increase risk of clotting
Dong quai	anticoagulants: additive effects may increase bleeding risk
Fish oil	anticoagulants: potentially increased bleeding risk antihypertensives: additive effects may further lower blood pressure lipid-lowering drugs: despite triglyceride-lowering effect, may antagonize drug by slightly increasing LDL-C levels
Folate	anti-seizure drugs: may decrease phenytoin absorption

(*Continued*)

Table 3.4 (*Continued*)

Dietary Supplement	Interaction(s)
Garlic	anticoagulants: may increase bleeding risk antihypertensives: potential additive effect, causing small reductions in blood pressure lipid-lowering drugs: potential additive effect on total cholesterol and LDL-C HIV drugs: may decrease effect of protease inhibitors
Ginger	anticoagulants: additive effects may increase bleeding risk cardiac glycosides: may increase or decrease drug effects
Ginkgo biloba	anticoagulants: additive effects may increase bleeding risk antihypertensives: additive effects may further reduce blood pressure thiazide diuretics: additive effects may further reduce blood pressure
Ginseng	diabetes drugs: may further lower blood glucose stimulant drugs: may increase drug effects
Kava	hypnotic drugs: may increase sedation of benzodiazepines
Melatonin	anticoagulants: may increase clotting risk antihypertensives: additive effects may further reduce blood pressure; may increase blood pressure when taken with calcium-channel blockers
Saw palmetto	anticoagulants: potentially increased bleeding risk antihypertensives: may increase blood pressure
St. John's wort	anticoagulants: may increase bleeding risk digoxin: may decrease drug concentration statin drugs: may decrease drug concentration indinavir: may decrease drug concentration antidepressants: may increase drug concentration
Vitamin E	anticoagulants: may increase bleeding risk

Note: This table is not all-inclusive. Information adapted from the Natural Standard (www.naturalstandard.com).

Interactions with Other Dietary Supplements

Although the potential for a dietary supplement to interact with others exists, currently there is not enough evidence to identify those risks. This should not be interpreted as there being no risk, however, only that none has been identified.

Potentially Dangerous Dietary Supplements

Several dietary supplements have been identified as more likely to cause harm than others. The FDA, the National Center on Complementary and Alternative Medicine, the consumer protection and education magazine *Consumer Reports*, and other organizations have published warnings for consumers (Table 3.5). Review of the scientific literature and actual adverse event reports revealed that these supplements may cause organ damage, cancer, or other adverse effects; are currently the subject of an FDA warning; or pose significant theoretical risks.

Dietary Supplement Verification Programs

Three organizations analyze dietary supplements to ensure safety, the U.S. Pharmacopeia (USP), ConsumerLab.com, and the Natural Products Association (NPA).

The USP is an independent, nonprofit organization that establishes standards for all prescription and over-the-counter drugs, dietary supplements, and other healthcare products manufactured in the United States, such as medical devices. Founded in 1820, the USP is recognized by federal law as the official body that sets standards for drugs and dietary

Table 3.5 Potentially Hazardous Dietary Supplements

Dietary Supplement	Status	Effects
Androstenedione (also known as "andro")	banned in other countries, FDA has issued a warning, or adverse effects are shown in studies	may alter levels of sex hormones; may increase risk of some cancers; may affect growth in children and adolescents
Aristolochic acid	documented organ failure and known carcinogenic properties	may cause kidney disease and urothelial cancer
Bitter orange	adverse events reported or theoretical risks identified	may cause ventricular arrhythmias, increased heart rate, and cardiac arrest
Chaparral	banned in other counties, FDA has issued a warning, or adverse effects are shown in studies	may cause liver damage
Comfrey	banned in other counties, FDA has issued a warning, or adverse effects are shown in studies	may obstruct blood flow to the liver; may increase risk of some cancers
Dieter's teas	adverse events reported or theoretical risks identified	may cause excessive laxative effect and electrolyte imbalance
Ephedra	adverse events reported and removed from U.S. market	heart palpitations, seizure, heart attack, stroke, death
Germander	banned in other countries, FDA has issued a warning, or adverse effects are shown in studies	may cause liver damage

(Continued)

Table 3.5 (*Continued*)

Dietary Supplement	Status	Effects
GHB (gamma hydroxybutyric acid), GBL (gamma butyrolactone), and BD (1,4-butanediol)	FDA has issued a warning	may decrease breathing rate; may cause vomiting, seizures, coma, and death
Kava	banned in other counties, FDA has issued a warning, or adverse effects are shown in studies	may cause liver disease and liver failure
L-tryptophan	adverse events reported	may cause eosinophilia myalgia syndrome
Lobelia	adverse events reported or theoretical risks identified	may stimulate or depress the nervous system; may increase or decrease breathing rate
Niacin	adverse events reported or theoretical risks identified	may cause liver toxicity; may alter blood sugar and uric acid levels; may worsen stomach ulcers

Table 3.5 (*Continued*)

Dietary Supplement	Status	Effects
Organ/glandular extracts (animal)	adverse events reported or theoretical risks identified	may be contaminated; may communicate animal diseases (mad cow disease)
PC SPES, SPES, and skullcap	FDA has issued a warning	may contain undeclared prescription drugs (warfarin and alprazolam)
Pennyroyal oil	adverse events reported or theoretical risks identified	may cause seizures
Yohimbe	adverse events reported or theoretical risks identified	may lower blood pressure; may cause kidney damage; may cause anxiety
Vitamin A	adverse events shown in studies	vitamin A toxicity (headache, fatigue, dizziness, blurry vision, bone pain, nausea and/or vomiting); may cause liver damage

Note: This table is not all-inclusive. Adverse effects are more likely to occur if an individual consumes a dietary supplement with known dangers or uses more than the recommended dose (as exposure to too much of any biologically active component may cause harm).
FDA, Food and Drug Administration.

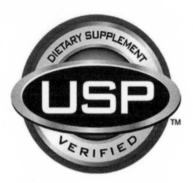

Figure 3.1 Mark of the U.S. Pharmocopeia. Reprinted with permission from the U.S. Pharmocopeia © 2006.

supplements. The USP aims to improve public health by ensuring the high quality of drugs and dietary supplements by setting high standards and working with various entities, including manufacturers and healthcare providers, to meet those standards.

While drug manufacturers must comply with USP standards, manufacturers of dietary supplements voluntarily participate in the relatively new USP verification program (launched in October 2001), which consists of independent, third-party testing and evaluation of ingredients used in dietary supplements and the finished products. The USP verification program for dietary supplements is based on the use of current good manufacturing practices.

The USP also created a mark (Fig. 3.1) that can be placed on packaging of products that meet their specific standards. The USP mark tells you that the product contains tested and verified ingredients and final product and that manufacturing processes meet established standards. Dietary supplements bearing the USP mark contain the ingredients stated on the label; contain the ingredients in the amounts stated on the label; will be metabolized to release the nutrients for absorption in the body; have been screened for harmful levels of contaminants, including pesticides, bacteria, and heavy metals; and have been manufactured using safe, sanitary, and controlled procedures.

The USP currently verifies vitamin and mineral supplements and is in the process of continually adding similar information for herbal, botanical, and other dietary supplements. The USP web site (http://www.usp.org) provides detailed information regarding the exact brands and specific types of dietary supplements that have been evaluated and meet USP standards for purity, dissolution, and manufacturing. There is also a directory of where such dietary supplements can be purchased. For a list of current USP-verified dietary supplement manufacturers and brands, see Appendix C.

ConsumerLab.com conducts independent product reviews of multiple brands of dietary supplements claiming to contain the same key ingredient (such as *Gingko biloba*). These product reviews are conducted every 24 to 36 months for each product category and include the results of blinded tests performed by academic and commercial labs that Consumer-Lab.com selects. Results are posted on their web site (http://www.ConsumerLab.com) for online subscribers, and free general information is also available. By paying a testing fee, dietary supplement manufacturers and distributors may choose to participate in the Voluntary Certification Program of ConsumerLab.com. Brands that meet the standards for identity, strength, purity, and pill disintegration are posted on the ConsumerLab.com web site and may be licensed to carry the Approved Quality Products Seal shown in Figure 3.2. In order to continue to carry the seal, those products must be retested every 12 months to ensure consistency. The seal indicates that a product meets recognized standards of quality,

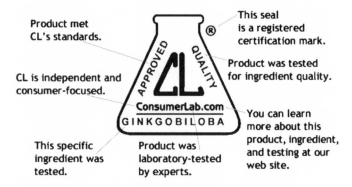

Figure 3.2 ConsumerLab.com approved quality seal. Reprinted with permission from ConsumerLab.com © 2006.

contains the quantity of ingredients stated on the label, is free of contaminants, and breaks apart properly so that it can be absorbed.

The NPA (www.naturalproductassoc.org), formerly known as the National Nutritional Foods Association, is a nonprofit organization that protects consumers and manufacturers by ensuring product quality and label integrity in the dietary supplement industry. The NPA modeled its own Good Manufacturing Practices Certification Program after the GMPs recommended by members of the dietary supplement industry in 1997. This program consists of random third-party inspections of members' manufacturing facilities to determine whether they meet specifications for staff training, cleanliness, equipment maintenance, record keeping, and handling of raw materials. The NPA's TruLabel Program randomly tests members' products for "label integrity" to ensure that the product contents are as listed. Members of the NPA that manufacture dietary supplements under their own label have been required to participate in this program since 1990.

4. Deconstructing Dietary Supplements

What makes understanding and regulating dietary supplements so complex is that many different substances are lumped together in one group. Dr. Jeffrey Blumberg, senior scientist and director of the Antioxidants Laboratory at the Human Nutrition Research Center on Aging at Tufts University, contends that including all of these different substances under one heading is "worse than comparing apples with oranges."

As discussed in chapter 2, dietary supplements are not foods, but they are regulated in a way that is closest to the way the FDA regulates foods. They are not drugs, but they are marketed in ways that are similar to some over-the-counter and prescription drugs. For the purposes of this chapter, I have divided dietary supplements into vitamin and mineral supplements, herbal and botanical supplements, and other supplements.

Vitamin and Mineral Dietary Supplements

Table 4.1 lists the vitamins according to whether they are fat- or water-soluble. Those minerals necessary for a healthy diet are boron, calcium, chromium, copper, iodine, iron, magnesium, manganese, phosphorus, potassium, selenium, and zinc. To prevent illness and death from vitamin and mineral deficiencies, the U.S. government established the recommended dietary allowances (RDAs) in 1943. These values are

Table 4.1 The Vitamins

Fat-soluble	vitamin A
	vitamin D
	vitamin E
	vitamin K
Water-soluble	vitamin B_1 (thiamin)
	vitamin B_2 (riboflavin)
	vitamin B_3 (niacin)
	vitamin B_6 (pyridoxine)
	vitamin B_{12} (cobalamine)
	vitamin C
	folate
	pantothenic acid
	biotin
	choline
	inositol
	PABA

updated routinely based on new scientific information. Recently, dietary reference intakes (DRIs) were established by the Institute of Medicine's Food and Nutrition Board to recommend how much of various nutrients individuals and groups of people should be consuming, not just to avoid deficiency but also to optimize health. Continuing efforts are made to explore the possibility that even higher amounts of certain nutrients may provide additional health benefits. To establish the DRIs, experts in nutrition, dietetics, statistics, nutrition epidemiology, public health, economics, and consumer perceptions reviewed the scientific evidence of safety, efficacy, toxicity, and beneficial properties of vitamins, minerals, and a few non-vitamin/non-mineral substances such as water and fiber. The DRIs are listed in Appendix A.

The DRIs are nutrient-based reference values that include an estimated average requirement (EAR) and an RDA. When

Table 4.2 Dietary Reference Intakes

Measure	Definition
Estimated Average Requirement (EAR)	the average daily nutrient intake level estimated to meet the requirement of half the healthy individuals in a particular life stage and gender group
Recommended Dietary Allowance (RDA)	the average daily nutrient intake level sufficient to meet the nutrient requirement of nearly all (97–98%) healthy individuals in a particular life stage and gender group
Adequate Intake (AI)	a recommended average daily nutrient intake level based on observed or experimentally determined approximations of estimates of nutrient intake by a group (or groups) of healthy people that are assumed to be adequate; used when an RDA cannot be determined
Tolerable Upper Intake Level (UL)	the highest average daily nutrient intake level likely to pose no risk of adverse health effects to almost all individuals in a particular life stage and gender group; as intake increases above the UL, the potential risk of adverse health effects increases

Adapted from Dietary Reference Intakes, Applications in Dietary Planning, Institute of Medicine, 2003.

there is not enough information to determine an EAR and an RDA, an adequate intake (AI) is established. Many nutrients also have a tolerable upper intake level (UL). The values in Table 4.2 were established to guide the consumption of a complete and nutritious diet. Vitamin and mineral dietary supplements may contain a single nutrient (such as vitamin C) or multiple nutrients (such as B-complex or multivitamins). Doses of vitamins and minerals in dietary supplements vary from levels close to the RDA or AI to several times those levels.

The DRIs are used to provide food-based dietary guidance; they are accompanied by national food guides and dietary guidelines for healthy people and provide a basis for food and dietary supplement labels. Although the DRIs and the accompanying guidelines (such as the *Dietary Guidelines for Americans* and the *Food Guide Pyramid*) specify daily goals, health professionals use these tools to help people choose diets that provide the recommended nutrients over time.

Several false assumptions have been made regarding vitamin and mineral dietary supplements. For example, vitamin A deficiency causes decreased night vision and, if very severe, blindness. Treating deficient individuals with vitamin A may indeed improve vision. However, many dietary supplements containing vitamin A and beta-carotene (a precursor to vitamin A) claim to "support good eye health." Some consumers falsely assume that if the deficiency of a vitamin or mineral harms a system or organ, then consuming that vitamin or mineral when the body is not in a deficient state will strengthen that system or organ. Some additional assumptions regarding vitamin and mineral dietary supplements are listed in Table 4.3.

Much of the research on vitamins and minerals has investigated whether dietary supplements are superior to food. According to two recent scientific publications by Dr. Alice H. Lichtenstein and Dr. Robert M. Russell, both from the Human Nutrition Research Center on Aging at Tufts University, the answer is no. However, most experts do agree that further research is worth pursuing.

Herbal and Botanical Dietary Supplements

Herbal and botanical dietary supplements have been used as medicines for thousands of years. For example, black

Table 4.3 Assumptions Made Regarding Vitamin and Mineral Dietary Supplements

Assumption	Reality	Examples
If some is good, more is better.	Fat-soluble vitamins are stored in the body. Intake of fat-soluble vitamins that exceeds the established tolerable upper intake level can have serious negative affects.	Excessive intake of vitamin K can interfere with certain medications that affect blood clotting. Excessive consumption of vitamin A may cause toxicity and liver damage.
Water-soluble vitamins are excreted so they must be safe.	There are exceptions to this generality.	Mega-doses of vitamin C, a popular but ineffective cold remedy, can cause diarrhea and gastrointestinal distress. Intake of vitamin B_6 at levels several times the tolerable upper intake level may cause neurologic symptoms such as numbness, tingling, bone pain, and muscle weakness.
Antioxidants must be safe and health-promoting.	Although intake of antioxidants is associated with decreased incidence of chronic diseases, including heart disease and cancer, there is little evidence to support taking more than the established levels and effects of high consumption may vary among individuals.	A recent study examining high intakes of vitamin E from supplements and heart disease showed that supplementation might have increased the incidence of stroke. Two separate studies evaluating the cancer-preventing power of beta-carotene showed that it actually increased the incidence of lung cancer in smokers.

cohosh (*Cimicifuga racemosa*), which is now commonly used to relieve symptoms associated with menopause, was used by Native Americans for a variety of ailments. They boiled black cohosh root in water and drank the resulting beverage for health problems ranging from rheumatism and sore throat to "diseases of women" and "debility." As far back as 5000 years ago, ephedra (ma huang, *Ephedra sinica*) was used in China and India to treat bronchial asthma and related ailments. Many cultures around the world continue to make use of herbs and botanicals for medicinal purposes.

Historic and anecdotal information and scientific data suggest that herbal and botanical dietary supplements have a high level of biologic activity and, in many cases, act as medicines. Despite their widespread use over time, however, scientific evidence supporting their efficacy and safety is lacking. Nevertheless, many herbal remedies are among the most popular dietary supplements purchased and used regularly in the United States. Table 4.4 lists some of these herbal and

Table 4.4 Some Popular Herbal and Botanical Dietary Supplements

Alfalfa	Goldenseal
Black cohosh	Green tea (green tea extract)
Burdock	Kava
Dandelion	Melatonin
Dong quai	Saw palmetto
Echinacea	Skullcap
Evening primrose	Soy (soy protein)
Flaxseed	Spirulina
Garlic	St. John's wort
Ginger	Valerian
Ginkgo biloba	Whey protein
Ginseng	Yohimbe

botanical dietary supplements, but the information is by no means all-inclusive.

Based on historic uses, several assumptions have been made regarding herbal and botanical dietary supplements, despite a lack of scientific evidence. For example, ginseng (*Panax ginseng*), which can have an unusual and almost human appearance, is recommended for common ailments such as lack of energy, lagging libido, and a poor immune system.

In addition, many herbal and botanical dietary supplements are promoted for uses that are unsupported or have been disproved. Comfrey (*Symphytum officinale*) has been and continues to be used for a variety of conditions associated with inflammation, including diseases of the gastrointestinal and respiratory system. No evidence supports these uses, however, and comfrey is among the herbal and botanical dietary supplements currently considered extremely dangerous. Another very popular herbal remedy, echinacea (*Echinacea purpurea, Echinacea angustifolia*), has been shown in three scientific studies to be ineffective at preventing or decreasing the severity of the common cold.

Perhaps the most common assumption about herbal and botanical dietary supplements is that one name refers to one "herbal medicine." In truth, there are so many common names and parts of various plants that are used that it is sometimes impossible to identify exactly what is encapsulated in an herbal or botanical dietary supplement. Kelp, which is used in folk medicine to treat constipation, bronchitis, emphysema, asthma, indigestion, ulcers, colitis, gallstones, obesity, and genitourinary and reproductive abnormalities in both men and women, actually refers to a huge family of seaweeds and algae. It is extremely difficult to evaluate the efficacy of a substance whose origin cannot be identified.

Other Dietary Supplements

Vitamins and minerals share the quality of being highly
studied and classified dietary components, and herbal and
botanical dietary supplements are all used as natural medicines.
Other dietary supplements are alike in that they elude such
organization. Essentially categorized by default, some of the
dietary supplements in this group (Table 4.5) are components
of plants (such as flavonoids), some are found in animal sources
(such as fish oil), and others are already present in small quantities in our bodies (such as coenzyme Q10, glutathione, and
L-carnitine). Most are available through eating foods, such as
fruits, vegetables, grains, nuts, seeds, and animal protein
sources.

The evidence of activity for these substances when isolated
in a dietary supplement, however, is highly variable. Some of
these dietary supplements have very little scientific evidence
to support their use, while others have a strong scientific basis
for their use. L-carnitine, for example, has been promoted for
use in cardiovascular disease, neurological diseases, depressed
immunity, and obesity, but its efficacy lacks sufficient high-
quality evidence from mainstream scientific studies. In contrast, dietary supplements containing chondroitin sulfate,

Table 4.5 Some Popular Other Dietary Supplements

Alpha-lipoic acid	Fish oil
Chitosan	Flavonoids
Chondroitan-sulfate	Glucosamine
Coenzyme Q10	Glutathione
Creatine	L-carnitine
DHEA	N-acetylcysteine
Essential fatty acids	Shark cartilage

which can be found in shark, beef cartilage, or bovine trachea, have been the subject of numerous well-controlled studies and have been found to significantly improve osteoarthritis.

As more information becomes available regarding members of this group of dietary supplements, we may be able to better categorize them. For now, however, each dietary supplement in this broad category must be considered independently.

Evidence of Dietary Supplement Efficacy

The Natural Standard is composed of a panel of experts, including medical doctors, pharmacists, and those working in the fields of medicine, nutrition, complementary and alternative therapies, and dietary supplements. The Natural Standard (http://www.naturalstandard.com) provides a clearinghouse of the vast research performed on various vitamin, mineral, herbal, botanical, and other dietary supplements. The group classifies dietary supplements and their specific uses based on extensive reviews of the scientific literature, and these reports are evaluated by experts and reviewed by their peers. The methods used are based on currently accepted and rigorous scientific standards. Table 4.6 explains this classification system further.

Omega-3 fatty acids such as those found in fish oil are a popular dietary supplement with several purported effects. To evaluate the existing literature on omega-3 fatty acids, the Natural Standard reviewed 252 individual references, most of which were from peer-reviewed journals. Based on the quality (the types of studies available and how many are randomized, controlled trials) and quantity (the number of randomized, controlled trials available) of evidence, the Natural Standard determined that there was "strong scientific evidence" (level A)

Table 4.6 Natural Standard's Approach to Classifying Dietary Supplements Based on Scientific Evidence

Level of evidence	Classification	Scientific Basis
A	strong scientific evidence	Evidence of a benefit has been found in more than two RCTs **or** Evidence of a benefit has been found in one RCT and one review of multiple studies (also known as a meta-analysis) **or** Multiple RCTs have been done and a majority suggest a benefit of the dietary supplement **and** evidence from other information supports this benefit
B	good scientific evidence	Evidence of a benefit has been found in one or two RCTs **or** Evidence of a benefit has been found in one or more analyses of multiple studies **or** Evidence of a benefit has been found in one or more less well-controlled studies **and** other information supports this benefit
C	unclear or conflicting scientific evidence	Evidence of a benefit from one or more small RCTs **or** Conflicting evidence from several RCTs without adequate suggestion of a benefit **or** Evidence of a benefit from one or more less well-controlled trials **and** suggestion of no benefit from other sources of information **or** Evidence of a benefit only from other sources of information, such as basic science, animal research, or scientific theory
D	fair negative scientific evidence	Evidence of no benefit from one or more less well-controlled trials **and** other information supports this lack of benefit
F	strong negative scientific evidence	Evidence of no benefit from one or more RCTs
	lack of evidence	Inadequate research on humans to evaluate a dietary supplement

Reprinted with permission from Natural Standard. © 2006 (www.naturalstandard.com). RCT, randomized controlled trial.

for the use of omega-3 fatty acids in lowering triglycerides, a component of blood cholesterol. In addition, the group determined that there was "good scientific evidence" (level B) for the use of omega-3 fatty acids (in the form of fish oil) for alleviation of morning stiffness and joint tenderness of rheumatoid arthritis. Table 4.7 lists dietary supplements with strong scientific evidence of a positive effect or of having no effect.

Table 4.7 Dietary Supplements with Strong Scientific Evidence of a Positive Effect or No Effect

Dietary Supplement	Condition	Evidence*
Aloe vera	constipation	A
Andrographis paniculata Nees, Kan Jang, SHA-10	upper respiratory infection	A
Arginine	Food and Drug Administration-approved growth hormone/pituitary/ urea disorders treatment	A
	asthma	F
Beta-carotene	erythropoietic protoporphyria (painful skin sensitivity to sunlight)	A
Beta-glucan	high cholesterol	A
Beta-sitosterol	high cholesterol	A
Biotin	biotin deficiency	A
Calcium	antacid	A
	osteoporosis prevention	A
	calcium deficiency	A
	high blood phosphorus levels	A
	magnesium toxicity	A
Chondroitin sulfate	osteoarthritis	A

(*Continued*)

Table 4.7 (*Continued*)

Dietary Supplement	Condition	Evidence*
Copper	copper deficiency	A
Ephedra	weight loss	A
Fish oil	high blood pressure	A
	high triglycerides	A
	secondary heart disease prevention	A
Folate	folate deficiency	A
	megaloblastic anemia	A
	prevention of neural tube defects	A
	fragile X syndrome	F
Ginkgo biloba	claudication	A
	dementia	A
Glucosamine	mild to moderate osteoarthritis of the knee	A
Hawthorne	congestive heart failure	A
Horse chestnut	chronic venous insufficiency	A
Inositol	high cholesterol	A
	pellagra	A
Iodine	goiter prevention	A
	iodine deficiency	A
	radiation emergency	A
	skin disinfectant	A
	water purification	A
	iodine deficiency	A
Iron	iron-deficiency anemia	A
	anemia of chronic disease	A
Kava	anxiety	A
Melatonin	jet lag	A
Niacin	high cholesterol	A
	pellagra (niacin deficiency)	A

(*Continued*)

Table 4.7 (*Continued*)

Dietary Supplement	Condition	Evidence*
Pantothenic acid	pantothenic acid deficiency	A
Phosphorus/phosphates	constipation	A
	high blood calcium levels	A
	low blood phosphorus levels	A
	kidney stones	A
Policosanol	high cholesterol	A
	platelet aggregation	A
Probiotics	Helicobacter pylori infection	A
Psyllium	high cholesterol	A
Red yeast rice	high cholesterol	A
Riboflavin	riboflavin deficiency	A
	jaundice in the newborn	A
Saw palmetto	benign prostatic hyperplasia	A
Soy	high cholesterol	A
St. John's wort	mild to moderate depression	A
Thiamin	thiamin deficiency	A
Vitamin A (retinol)	acne	A
	acute promyelocytic leukemia	A
	measles	A
	vitamin A deficiency	A
	xeropthalmia	A
Vitamin B_6	hereditary sideroblastic anemia	A
	prevention of adverse effects in people taking cycloserine	A
	vitamin B_6 deficiency	A
	pyridoxine-dependent seizures in newborns	A
Vitamin B_{12}	vitamin B_{12} deficiency	A
	megaloblastic and pernicious anemia	A
	Leber's disease	F

(*Continued*)

Table 4.7 (*Continued*)

Dietary Supplement	Condition	Evidence*
Vitamin C	vitamin C deficiency/scurvy	A
Vitamin D	familial hypophosphatemia (poor calcium and phosphate absorption)	A
	Fanconi syndrome–related hypophosphatemia	A
	hyperparathyroidism secondary to low vitamin D levels	A
	hypocalcemia secondary to hypoparathyroidism	A
	osteomalacia	A
	psoriasis	A
	rickets	A
Vitamin E	vitamin E deficiency	A
Vitamin K	hemorrhagic disease of the newborn	A
	vitamin K deficiency	A
Zinc	diarrhea in children	A
	gastric ulcers	A
	sickle cell anemia	A

Reprinted with permission from Natural Standard. © 2006
(www.naturalstandard.com).
*A, positive effect; F, no effect.

5. Researching Dietary Supplements

Despite their natural connotation, dietary supplements are biologically active substances. Evidence for their safety and efficacy should therefore be based on accepted principles of science.

What Is Good Science?

The Agency for Healthcare Research and Quality ranked scientific studies by the value of their results. Below they are ranked from most powerful to least powerful:

- prospective, randomized, double-blind, placebo-controlled clinical trial with crossover;
- prospective, randomized, double-blind clinical trial;
- single-blind clinical trial;
- open-label clinical trial;
- retrospective epidemiological study;
- other types of consumer or patient-based, interview-type studies (including meta-analyses).

Randomized, controlled trials are considered the gold standard of scientific research. Such trials include a control group, people who are observed but receive no treatment of any kind, and an intervention group, people who receive a certain treatment, such as a dietary supplement. Members of the control and intervention groups are similar (matched) in age, sex, ethnicity, marital status, socioeconomic status, health status, and diet and are randomly assigned to the respective groups. The power of such a trial is that it controls for any variation between the two groups, so that the only relevant difference is that the intervention group receives the specific treatment. Thus, any difference in the outcomes between the control and intervention groups is likely attributable to the intervention.

To determine whether the results of a study are due to the intervention or to chance, scientists conduct statistical analyses. A P value (probability value) of 0.05 is generally used to indicate statistical significance. P values greater than 0.05 indicate that the likelihood the results were a product of chance is greater than 5 percent. Conversely, the smaller the P value, the more significant the results. Thus, a P value lower than 0.001 indicates that it is very unlikely the results were due to chance; that is, the intervention had a highly significant effect on the treatment group.

In case-control studies, cases who have a particular outcome (for example, a disease) are identified and their past exposure to various components (such as a dietary supplement) is compared with that of control subjects, who do not have the particular outcome. By matching case and control subjects for sex, age, and other variables, there is less chance that the results are due to anything but the difference in exposure.

Cross-sectional studies measure the prevalence of a health outcome (for example, a disease) or determinants of health (such as ethnicity) in a population at any one time. For example, a cross-sectional study could measure the relationship between osteoporosis and calcium intake. This type of study is vulnerable to confounding, however, as a result of selection bias, which distorts statistical analysis by including a sample that is not representative of the population of interest. In addition, cross-sectional studies are not good for determining cause and effect.

Cohort studies are long-term studies that compare subjects who have a particular outcome (for example, a disease) and/or who receive a particular intervention (such as a dietary supplement) with those who do not have that outcome or exposure. Cohort studies tend to be less reliable than randomized, controlled trials because there is less control over the differences between the two groups. For more accurate results, cohort studies may have to last for several years, which allows for additional differences between the groups to enter into the study and confound the results.

The validity of a scientific study should determine whether it is published in a prestigious scientific journal, such as the *Journal of the American Medical Association* and the *New England Journal of Medicine*. Most scientific journals require that published material is reviewed by peers, other experts who can evaluate the strength of the evidence and identify shortcomings of studies. Published studies can be retrieved online at PubMed (see Appendix D).

Many dietary supplement manufacturers promote their products through testimonials and anecdotes from satisfied customers. While persuasive, testimonials cannot replace scientific evidence and are often fabricated, paid for, or provided by people who are emotionally bound to a product. Testimonials should never be substituted for rigorous scientific data.

Who Are the Experts?

Consumers get information about dietary supplements from many sources, including friends, family members, and healthcare professionals. This information is often a mixture of scientific data, hearsay, and anecdote. Given the complexity of dietary supplements, however, only people with in-depth knowledge of science, medicine, and nutrition should be considered experts.

Registered dietitians, pharmacists, physicians, nurses, and physician assistants tend to be the most informed about the scientific evidence on dietary supplements. Registered dietitians are certified by the American Dietetic Association, and during the last several years, dietary supplements have become a major focus of their training and practice. In addition to answering specific questions about dietary supplements, a registered dietitian can determine individual nutrient needs based on age, sex, life stage (for instance, premenopausal versus postmenopausal women), and medical history. By analyzing the diet (including intake of fortified foods and dietary supplements), a registered dietitian can determine whether a person is consuming the recommended levels of nutrients or if any nutrients are lacking or being consumed in excess. Based on these results, a dietitian can recommend improvements to the diet and/or if dietary supplementation should be considered.

Pharmacists are trained to understand drug formulation and interactions. In addition to answering specific questions about dietary supplements, they can recognize potential interactions between dietary supplements and drugs. Pharmacists can also help identify those dietary supplements verified by the USP, ConsumerLab.com, or the NPA, as well as the recommended doses.

Physicians (MDs, DOs), nurses (RNs, NPs), and physician assistants are gradually becoming cognizant of the widespread use of dietary supplements. As a companion to the *Physician's Desk Reference*, an immense and detailed catalogue of drug and prescribing information that can be found in virtually any doctor's office or library, a new *Physicians Desk Reference for Nonprescription Drugs, Dietary Supplements, and Herbs* has been created. Physicians, nurses, and physician assistants can be useful resources regarding dietary supplements, including whether there is adequate evidence to support a benefit, no effect, or potential for harm.

People considering taking dietary supplements can benefit from consulting a knowledgeable expert. This is especially true for women who are breastfeeding or pregnant (or who may become pregnant); older individuals; people of smaller stature; people with chronic medical conditions such as cardiovascular disease, diabetes, or hypertension; and people with upcoming surgery. In addition, a pediatrician should be consulted when considering giving a dietary supplement to a child.

Dietary Supplement Information in the Media

Information about dietary supplements can also be found in books, magazines, newspapers, television shows, radio programs, and web sites, and these sources contain a range of reliable and unreliable information. Identifying accurate information should begin by determining the original source. If dietary supplement information does not come directly from an expert, it is important to establish whether an expert was consulted. (See Appendix D for a list of reliable resources on dietary supplements.)

Whether dietary supplement information is balanced, objective, and free of commercial influence can help determine if its motive is educational or promotional. Magazines and newspapers often contain full-page articles that seem to come from medical or scientific establishments;

upon closer examination, however, the word "advertisement" can often be found in small print at the top of the page, indicating that the information is indeed intended to sell something. Information contained in obvious advertisements can be misleading. Television commercials and lengthier infomercials are crafted so they appear to be backed by medical organizations. While these advertisements have the look and feel of a medical establishment, they are misleading and designed to sell a product to a vulnerable population.

Consider this common scenario: An attractive man or woman wearing a lab coat approaches the camera while speaking words of empathy to overweight viewers. "It's not your fault. You struggle with extra weight because of a malfunction in your body. *Dietary Supplement X* can reverse the effects of this malfunction and help you lose the extra pounds. Clinical trials have shown that people who take *Dietary Supplement X* lose weight faster and easier than those who do not take it." Inevitably, this monologue culminates in the opportunity to purchase *Dietary Supplement X*.

The format of information on dietary supplements can also provide cues as to its validity. Books, magazine and newspaper articles, and live newscasts deliver information in various levels of scope and depth. While a book might explore dietary supplements in great detail, a 60-second piece on the evening news might only offer tidbits that are sensational, very recent, or particularly interesting, without exploring the whole story. Shorter pieces, such as newspaper or magazine articles, may highlight the newest development regarding a dietary supplement but may not place this new information in context. Due to extended production and publication schedules, however, sources that do discuss dietary supplements in greater depth—such as books and encyclopedias—may not include the very latest information.

Dietary Supplement Research on the World Wide Web

The unique qualities of the World Wide Web can make it difficult to decipher reliable sources from poor ones. For example, a commercial web site may adopt the appearance of a scientifically based organization, with pictures of doctors and test tubes, references to clinical trials, graphics illustrating data, and alleged conclusions based on such data.

All web sites should clearly identify their purpose and source of funding. This information can usually be found at the bottom of the page or through a hyperlink labeled "About This Site" or "Mission." The web-site address can also provide some information: commercial web sites generally end in ".com," web sites affiliated with universities end in ".edu," and government-related web sites end in ".gov." Web-site addresses that end in ".org" or ".net" may be nonprofit or for-profit organizations. Advertisements featured on a specific web site might also allude to its motive.

The identity of a web site should always be clear. Because it is easy to link from one web site to another, it can be difficult for consumers to determine what site they are on and how they got there. Through a series of clicks, it is easy to navigate away from the original web site without noticing. For example, banner ads, which appear across the top of the web page, may show a calculator, such as one to calculate body mass index. However, when a consumer clicks on this ad to enter height and weight, he or she is redirected to a different web site that may or may not be affiliated with the previous one.

The date of material on the World Wide Web should also be clear. Responsible web-site operators regularly review and update their information to ensure accuracy. The date of the latest update can usually be found at the bottom of the web page. Information on web pages older than 3 to 6 months should be viewed as outdated.

Finally, how consumers are able to interact with a web site is important. At the bottom of most pages, you can contact the webmaster or web-site provider with questions or concerns. Web sites that ask you to sign in may do so to provide more tailored information or to sell your information to other commercial entities. Web sites may also contain "cookies" that track which other web sites you visit and use that information for commercial purposes.

Contacting Dietary Supplement Manufacturers

Contacting individual manufacturers can be the most efficient way to find specific information. The following is a list of important questions that can be asked of dietary supplement manufacturers.

- How can you prove the effectiveness and safety of your product?
- Can you share information with me about the tests you use to determine safety and effectiveness?
- What quality control systems do you have in place?
- How closely do you adhere to the FDA's current good manufacturing procedures?
- Can you provide educational materials that will help me to understand the evidence regarding your product?
- Have you received any reports of adverse events?

Spotting False Claims

The sheer volume of available dietary supplements makes it difficult for the FDA to monitor all of these products. It is important to recognize these limitations and become an informed consumer. Products making unrealistic statements, claiming to be all-natural and therefore harmless, or claiming to contain "ancient" or "secret" ingredients should be viewed with extreme caution.

As discussed in chapter 2, the DSHEA states that dietary supplements cannot be claimed to treat or cure disease and that doing so identifies the product as a drug. For example, manufacturers of coral calcium, a calcium supplement said to be derived from living coral reefs, claimed their product could be used to treat ailments ranging from cancer to lupus to multiple sclerosis. While the people making these statements have been contacted (and are prohibited by the Federal Trade Commission from claiming that coral calcium cures a range of diseases and/or is absorbed easier than other calcium supplements), dietary supplements violating this regulation continue to be available to consumers. Dietary supplement safety should be ascertained using multiple resources. While dietary supplement labels contain vital information for consumers, a lack of cautionary words on labels should not be considered a statement of absolute safety.

Even after a recall has been effected, there is a risk of consuming harmful substances in products still available for purchase. In addition, substances that belong to the same class as a recalled dietary supplement may cause similar effects. Bitter orange (*Citrus aurantium*), for example, mimics certain characteristics of ephedra. Now that ephedra-containing products have been removed from the U.S. market, bitter orange is commonly found in weight-loss dietary supplements.

In conclusion, each piece of information about dietary supplements should be considered another piece of data. Educated decisions based on information from a variety of sources allows consumers to place recent developments in the appropriate context. Information should be continually updated as new data become available.

Appendix A. Dietary Reference Intakes

Dietary Reference Intakes (DRIs): Recommended Intakes for Individuals, Vitamins

Food and Nutrition Board, Institute of Medicine, National Academies

Life Stage Group	Vit A (μg/d)[a]	Vit C (mg/d)	Vit D (μg/d)[b,c]	Vit E (mg/d)[d]	Vit K (μg/d)	Thiamin (mg/d)
Infants						
0–6 mo	400*	40*	5*	4*	2.0*	0.2*
7–12 mo	500*	50*	5*	5*	2.5*	0.3*
Children						
1–3 y	**300**	**15**	5*	**6**	30*	**0.5**
4–8 y	**400**	**25**	5*	**7**	55*	**0.6**
Males						
9–13 y	**600**	**45**	5*	**11**	60*	**0.9**
14–18 y	**900**	**75**	5*	**15**	75*	**1.2**
19–30 y	**900**	**90**	5*	**15**	120*	**1.2**
31–50 y	**900**	**90**	5*	**15**	120*	**1.2**
51–70 y	**900**	**90**	10*	**15**	120*	**1.2**
>70 y	**900**	**90**	15*	**15**	120*	**1.2**
Females						
9–13 y	**600**	**45**	5*	**11**	60*	**0.9**
14–18 y	**700**	**65**	5*	**15**	75*	**1.0**
19–30 y	**700**	**75**	5*	**15**	90*	**1.1**
31–50 y	**700**	**75**	5*	**15**	90*	**1.1**
51–70 y	**700**	**75**	10*	**15**	90*	**1.1**
>70 y	**700**	**75**	15*	**15**	90*	**1.1**
Pregnancy						
14–18 y	**750**	**80**	5*	**15**	75*	**1.4**
19–30 y	**770**	**85**	5*	**15**	90*	**1.4**
31–50 y	**770**	**85**	5*	**15**	90*	**1.4**
Lactation						
14–18 y	**1,200**	**115**	5*	**19**	75*	**1.4**
19–30 y	**1,300**	**120**	5*	**19**	90*	**1.4**
31–50 y	**1,300**	**120**	5*	**19**	90*	**1.4**

NOTE: This table (taken from the DRI reports, see www.nap.edu) presents Recommended Dietary Allowances (RDAs) in **bold type** and Adequate Intakes (AIs) in ordinary type followed by an asterisk (*). RDAs and AIs may both be used as goals for individual intake. RDAs are set to meet the needs of almost all (97 to 98 percent) individuals in a group. For healthy breastfed infants, the AI is the mean intake. The AI for other life stage and gender groups is believed to cover needs of all individuals in the group, but lack of data or uncertainty in the data prevent being able to specify with confidence the percentage of individuals covered by this intake.

[a]As retinol activity equivalents (*RAE*s). 1 *RAE* = 1 μg retinol, 12 mg β-carotene, 24 μg α-carotene, or 24 μg β-cryptoxanthin. The *RAE* for dietary provitamin A carotenoids is twofold greater than retinol equivalents (*RE*), whereas the *RAE* for preformed vitamin A is the same as RE.

[b]As cholecalciferol. 1 μg cholecalciferol = 40 IU vitamin D.

[c]In the absence of adequate exposure to sunlight.

[d]As α-tocopherol. α-Tocopherol includes *RRR*-α-tocopherol, the only form of α-tocopherol that occurs naturally in foods, and the *2R*-stereoisomeric forms of α-tocopherol (*RRR*-, *RSR*-, *RRS*-, and *RSS*-α-tocopherol) that occur in fortified foods and supplements. It does not include the *2S*-stereoisomeric forms of α-tocopherol (*SRR*-, *SSR*-, *SRS*-, and *SSS*-α-tocopherol), also found in fortified foods and supplements.

Ribo-flavin (mg/d)	Niacin (mg/d)[e]	Vit B$_6$ (mg/d)	Folate (μg/d)[f]	Vit B$_{12}$ (μg/d)	Pantothenic Acid (mg/d)	Biotin (μg/d)	Choline[g] (mg/d)
0.3*	2*	0.1*	65*	0.4*	1.7*	5*	125*
0.4*	4*	0.3*	80*	0.5*	1.8*	6*	150*
0.5	6	0.5	150	0.9	2*	8*	200*
0.6	8	0.6	200	1.2	3*	12*	250*
0.9	12	1.0	300	1.8	4*	20*	375*
1.3	16	1.3	400	2.4	5*	25*	550*
1.3	16	1.3	400	2.4	5*	30*	550*
1.3	16	1.3	400	2.4	5*	30*	550*
1.3	16	1.7	400	2.4[i]	5*	30*	550*
1.3	16	1.7	400	2.4[i]	5*	30*	550*
0.9	12	1.0	300	1.8	4*	20*	375*
1.0	14	1.2	400[i]	2.4	5*	25*	400*
1.1	14	1.3	400[i]	2.4	5*	30*	425*
1.1	14	1.3	400[i]	2.4	5*	30*	425*
1.1	14	1.5	400	2.4[h]	5*	30*	425*
1.1	14	1.5	400	2.4[h]	5*	30*	425*
1.4	18	1.9	600[j]	2.6	6*	30*	450*
1.4	18	1.9	600[j]	2.6	6*	30*	450*
1.4	18	1.9	600[j]	2.6	6*	30*	450*
1.6	17	2.0	500	2.8	7*	35*	550*
1.6	17	2.0	500	2.8	7*	35*	550*
1.6	17	2.0	500	2.8	7*	35*	550*

[e]As niacin equivalents (NE). 1 μg of niacin = 60 μg of tryptophan; 0–6 months = preformed niacin (not NE).

[f]As dietary folate equivalents (DFE). 1 DFE = 1 μg food folate = 0.6 μg of folic acid from fortified food or as a supplement consumed with food = 0.5 μg of a supplement taken on an empty stomach.

[g]Although AIs have been set for choline, there are few data to assess whether a dietary supply of choline is needed at all stages of the life cycle, and it may be that the choline requirement can be met by endogenous synthesis at some of these stages.

[h]Because 10 to 30 percent of older people may malabsorb food-bound B$_{12}$, it is advisable for those older than 50 years to meet their RDA mainly by consuming foods fortified with B$_{12}$ or a supplement containing B$_{12}$.

[i]In view of evidence linking folate intake with neural tube defects in the fetus, it is recommended that all women capable of becoming pregnant consume 400 μg from supplements or fortified foods in addition to intake of food folate from a varied diet.

[j]It is assumed that women will continue consuming 400 μg from supplements or fortified food until their pregnancy is confirmed and they enter prenatal care, which ordinarily occurs after the end of the periconceptional period—the critical time for formation of the neural tube.

Dietary Reference Intakes (DRIs): Recommended Intakes for Individuals, Elements

Food and Nutrition Board, Institute of Medicine, National Academies

Life Stage Group	Calcium (mg/d)	Chromium (µg/d)	Copper (µg/d)	Fluoride (mg/d)	Iodine (µg/d)	Iron (mg/d)	Magnesium (mg/d)
Infants							
0–6 mo	210*	0.2*	200*	0.01*	110*	0.27*	30*
7–12 mo	270*	5.5*	220*	0.5*	130*	11	75*
Children							
1–3 y	500*	11*	340	0.7*	90	7	80
4–8 y	800*	15*	440	1*	90	10	130
Males							
9–13 y	1,300*	25*	700	2*	120	8	240
14–18 y	1,300*	35*	890	3*	150	11	410
19–30 y	1,000*	35*	900	4*	150	8	400
31–50 y	1,000*	35*	900	4*	150	8	420
51–70 y	1,200*	30*	900	4*	150	8	420
>70 y	1,200*	30*	900	4*	150	8	420
Females							
9–13 y	1,300*	21*	700	2*	120	8	240
14–18 y	1,300*	24*	890	3*	150	15	360
19–30 y	1,000*	25*	900	3*	150	18	310
31–50 y	1,000*	25*	900	3*	150	18	320
51–70 y	1,200*	20*	900	3*	150	8	320
>70 y	1,200*	20*	900	3*	150	8	320
Pregnancy							
14–18 y	1,300*	29*	1,000	3*	220	27	400
19–30 y	1,000*	30*	1,000	3*	220	27	350
31–50 y	1,000*	30*	1,000	3*	220	27	360
Lactation							
14–18 y	1,300*	44*	1,300	3*	290	10	360
19–30 y	1,000*	45*	1,300	3*	290	9	310
31–50 y	1,000*	45*	1,300	3*	290	9	320

NOTE: This table presents Recommended Dietary Allowances (RDAs) in **bold type** and Adequate Intakes (AIs) in ordinary type followed by an asterisk (*). RDAs and AIs may both be used as goals for individual intake. RDAs are set to meet the needs of almost all (97 to 98 percent) individuals in a group. For healthy breastfed infants, the AI is the mean intake. The AI for other life stage and gender groups is believed to cover needs of all individuals in the group, but lack of data or uncertainty in the data prevent being able to specify with confidence the percentage of individuals covered by this intake.

Manganese (mg/d)	Molybdenum (µg/d)	Phosphorus (mg/d)	Selenium (µg/d)	Zinc (mg/d)	Potassium (g/d)	Sodium (g/d)	Chloride (g/d)
0.003*	2*	100*	15*	2*	0.4*	0.12*	0.18*
0.6*	3*	275*	20*	3	0.7*	0.37*	0.57*
1.2*	17	460	20	3	3.0*	1.0*	1.5*
1.5*	22	500	30	5	3.8*	1.2*	1.9*
1.9*	34	1,250	40	8	4.5*	1.5*	2.3*
2.2*	43	1,250	55	11	4.7*	1.5*	2.3*
2.3*	45	700	55	11	4.7*	1.5*	2.3*
2.3*	45	700	55	11	4.7*	1.5*	2.3*
2.3*	45	700	55	11	4.7*	1.3*	2.0*
2.3*	45	700	55	11	4.7*	1.2*	1.8*
1.6*	34	1,250	40	8	4.5*	1.5*	2.3*
1.6*	43	1,250	55	9	4.7*	1.5*	2.3*
1.8*	45	700	55	8	4.7*	1.5*	2.3*
1.8*	45	700	55	8	4.7*	1.5*	2.3*
1.8*	45	700	55	8	4.7*	1.3*	2.0*
1.8*	45	700	55	8	4.7*	1.2*	1.8*
2.0*	50	1,250	60	12	4.7*	1.5*	2.3*
2.0*	50	700	60	11	4.7*	1.5*	2.3*
2.0*	50	700	60	11	4.7*	1.5*	2.3*
2.6*	50	1,250	70	13	5.1*	1.5*	2.3*
2.6*	50	700	70	12	5.1*	1.5*	2.3*
2.6*	50	700	70	12	5.1*	1.5*	2.3*

SOURCES: *Dietary Reference Intakes for Calcium, Phosphorous, Magnesium, Vitamin D, and Fluoride* (1997); *Dietary Reference Intakes for Thiamin, Riboflavin, Niacin, Vitamin B$_6$, Folate, Vitamin B$_{12}$, Pantothenic Acid, Biotin, and Choline* (1998); *Dietary Reference Intakes for Vitamin C, Vitamin E, Selenium, and Carotenoids* (2000); *Dietary Reference Intakes for Vitamin A, Vitamin K, Arsenic, Boron, Chromium, Copper, Iodine, Iron, Manganese, Molybdenum, Nickel, Silicon, Vanadium, and Zinc* (2001); and *Dietary Reference Intakes for Water, Potassium, Sodium, Chloride, and Sulfate* (2004). These reports may be accessed via http://www.nap.edu.

Appendix B. Dietary Supplement Health and Education Act

Public Law 103-417 103rd Congress

An Act

To amend the Federal Food, Drug, and Cosmetic Act to establish standards with respect to dietary supplements, and for other purposes.

Be it enacted by the Senate and House of Representatives of the United States of America in Congress assembled,

§1. Short Title; Reference; Table of Contents.

- **(a) Short Title.**
This Act may be cited as the "Dietary Supplement Health and Education Act of 1994".

- **(b) Reference.**
Whenever in this Act an amendment or repeal is expressed in terms of an amendment to, or repeal of, a section or other provision, the reference shall be considered to be made to a section or other provision of the Federal Food, Drug, and Cosmetic Act.

- **(c) Table of Contents.**
The table of contents of this Act is as follows:
Sec. 1. Short title; reference; table of contents.
Sec. 2. Findings.

Sec. 3. Definitions.
Sec. 4. Safety of dietary supplements and burden of proof
on FDA.
Sec. 5. Dietary supplement claims.
Sec. 6. Statements of nutritional support.
Sec. 7. Dietary supplement ingredient labeling and nutrition
information labeling.
Sec. 8. New dietary ingredients.
Sec. 9. Good manufacturing practices.
Sec. 10. Conforming amendments.
Sec. 11. Withdrawal of the regulations and notice.
Sec. 12. Commission on dietary supplement labels.
Sec. 13. Office of dietary supplements.

§2. Findings.

Congress finds that—

- (1) improving the health status of United States citizens ranks
  at the top of the national priorities of the Federal Government;
- (2) the importance of nutrition and the benefits of dietary
  supplements to health promotion and disease prevention
  have been documented increasingly in scientific studies;
- (3)(A) there is a link between the ingestion of certain nutrients or dietary supplements and the prevention of chronic
  diseases such as cancer, heart disease, and osteoporosis; and
- (B) clinical research has shown that several chronic diseases
  can be prevented simply with a healthful diet, such as a diet
  that is low in fat, saturated fat, cholesterol, and sodium,
  with a high proportion of plant-based foods;
- (4) healthful diets may mitigate the need for expensive medical
  procedures, such as coronary bypass surgery or angioplasty;

- (5) preventive health measures, including education, good nutrition, and appropriate use of safe nutritional supplements will limit the incidence of chronic diseases, and reduce long-term health care expenditures;
- (6)(A) promotion of good health and healthy lifestyles improves and extends lives while reducing health care expenditures; and
- (B) reduction in health care expenditures is of paramount importance to the future of the country and the economic well-being of the country;
- (7) there is a growing need for emphasis on the dissemination of information linking nutrition and long-term good health;
- (8) consumers should be empowered to make choices about preventive health care programs based on data from scientific studies of health benefits related to particular dietary supplements;
- (9) national surveys have revealed that almost 50 percent of the 260,000,000 Americans regularly consume dietary supplements of vitamins, minerals, or herbs as a means of improving their nutrition;
- (10) studies indicate that consumers are placing increased reliance on the use of nontraditional health care providers to avoid the excessive costs of traditional medical services and to obtain more holistic consideration of their needs;
- (11) the United States will spend over $1,000,000,000,000,000 on health care in 1994, which is about 12 percent of the Gross National Product of the United States, and this amount and percentage will continue to increase unless significant efforts are undertaken to reverse the increase;
- (12)(A) the nutritional supplement industry is an integral part of the economy of the United States;
- (B) the industry consistently projects a positive trade balance; and

- (C) the estimated 600 dietary supplement manufacturers in the United States produce approximately 4,000 products, with total annual sales of such products alone reaching at least $4,000,000,000;
- (13) although the Federal Government should take swift action against products that are unsafe or adulterated, the Federal Government should not take any actions to impose unreasonable regulatory barriers limiting or slowing the flow of safe products and accurate information to consumers;
- (14) dietary supplements are safe within a broad range of intake, and safety problems with the supplements are relatively rare; and
- (15)(A) legislative action that protects the right of access of consumers to safe dietary supplements is necessary in order to promote wellness; and
- (B) a rational Federal framework must be established to supersede the current ad hoc, patchwork regulatory policy on dietary supplements.

§3. Definitions.

- **(a) Definition of Certain Foods as Dietary Supplements.** Section 201 (21 U.S.C. 321) is amended by adding at the end the following:

  "(ff) The term "dietary supplement"—
    ○ "(1) means a product (other than tobacco) intended to supplement the diet that bears or contains one or more of the following dietary ingredients:
      ▪ "(A) a vitamin;
      ▪ "(B) a mineral;
      ▪ "(C) an herb or other botanical;
      ▪ "(D) an amino acid;

- "(E) a dietary substance for use by man to supplement the diet by increasing the total dietary intake; or
- "(F) a concentrate, metabolite, constituent, extract, or combination of any ingredient described in clause (A), (B), (C), (D), or (E);

○ "(2) means a product that—

- "(A)(i) is intended for ingestion in a form described in section 411(c)(1)(B)(i); or
- "(ii) complies with section 411(c)(1)(B)(ii);
- "(B) is not represented for use as a conventional food or as a sole item of a meal or the diet; and
- "(C) is labeled as a dietary supplement; and

○ "(3) does—

- "(A) include an article that is approved as a new drug under section 505, certified as an antibiotic under section 507, or licensed as a biologic under section 351 of the Public Health Service Act (42 U.S.C. 262) and was, prior to such approval, certification, or license, marketed as a dietary supplement or as a food unless the Secretary has issued a regulation, after notice and comment, finding that the article, when used as or in a dietary supplement under the conditions of use and dosages set forth in the labeling for such dietary supplement, is unlawful under section 402(f); and
- "(B) not include—
  - "(i) an article that is approved as a new drug under section 505, certified as an antibiotic under section 507, or

licensed as a biologic under section 351 of the Public Health Service Act (42 U.S.C. 262), or

- "(ii) an article authorized for investigation as a new drug, antibiotic, or biological for which substantial clinical investigations have been instituted and for which the existence of such investigations has been made public,

which was not before such approval, certification, licensing, or authorization marketed as a dietary supplement or as a food unless the Secretary, in the Secretary's discretion, has issued a regulation, after notice and comment, finding that the article would be lawful under this Act."

Except for purposes of section 201(g), a dietary supplement shall be deemed to be a food within the meaning of this Act.

- **(b) Exclusion from Definition of Food Additive.** Section 201(s) (21 U.S.C. 321(s)) is amended—
  - (1) by striking "or" at the end of subparagraph (4);
  - (2) by striking the period at the end of subparagraph (5) and inserting "; or"; and
  - (3) by adding at the end the following new subparagraph (6) "an ingredient described in paragraph (ff) in, or intended for use in, a dietary supplement.".
- **(c) Form of Ingestion.** Section 411(c)(1)(B) (21 U.S.C. 350(c)(1)(B)) is amended—
  - (1) in clause (i), by inserting "powder, softgel, gelcap," after "capsule,"; and
  - (2) in clause (ii), by striking "does not simulate and".

§4. Safety of Dietary Supplements and Burden of Proof on FDA.

Section 402 (21 U.S.C. 342) is amended by adding at the end the following:

- "(f)(1) If it is a dietary supplement or contains a dietary ingredient that—
  - "(A) presents a significant or unreasonable risk of illness or injury under—
    - "(i) conditions of use recommended or suggested in labeling, or
    - "(ii) if no conditions of use are suggested or recommended in the labeling, under ordinary conditions of use;
  - "(B) is a new dietary ingredient for which there is inadequate information to provide reasonable assurance that such ingredient does not present a significant or unreasonable risk of illness or injury;
  - "(C) the Secretary declares to pose an imminent hazard to public health or safety, except that the authority to make such declaration shall not be delegated and the Secretary shall promptly after such a declaration initiate a proceeding in accordance with sections 554 and 556 of title 5, United States Code, to affirm or withdraw the declaration; or
  - "(D) is or contains a dietary ingredient that renders it adulterated under paragraph (a)(1) under the conditions of use recommended or suggested in the labeling of such dietary supplement.
In any proceeding under this subparagraph, the United States shall bear the burden of proof on each element to

show that a dietary supplement is adulterated. The court shall decide any issue under this paragraph on a de novo basis.

- (2) Before the Secretary may report to a United States attorney a violation of paragraph (1)(A) for a civil proceeding, the person against whom such proceeding would be initiated shall be given appropriate notice and the opportunity to present views, orally and in writing, at least 10 days before such notice, with regard to such proceeding.

§5. Dietary Supplement Claims.

Chapter IV (21 U.S.C. 341 et seq.) is amended by inserting after section 403A the following new section:

DIETARY SUPPLEMENT LABELING EXEMPTIONS

- "Sec. 403B. (a) IN GENERAL.—A publication, including an article, a chapter in a book, or an official abstract of a peer-reviewed scientific publication that appears in an article and was prepared by the author or the editors of the publication, which is reprinted in its entirety, shall not be defined as labeling when used in connection with the sale of a dietary supplement to consumers when it—

    - "(1) is not false or misleading;
    - "(2) does not promote a particular manufacturer or brand of a dietary supplement;
    - "(3) is displayed or presented, or is displayed or presented with other such items on the same subject

matter, so as to present a balanced view of the available scientific information on a dietary supplement;

- ○ "(4) if displayed in an establishment, is physically separate from the dietary supplements; and
- ○ "(5) does not have appended to it any information by sticker or any other method.

- "(b) APPLICATION.—Subsection (a) shall not apply to or restrict a retailer or wholesaler of dietary supplements in any way whatsoever in the sale of books or other publications as a part of the business of such retailer or wholesaler.

- "(c) BURDEN OF PROOF.—In any proceeding brought under subsection (a), the burden of proof shall be on the United States to establish that an article or other such matter is false or misleading.".

§6. Statements of Nutritional Support.

Section 403(r) (21 U.S.C. 343(r)) is amended by adding at the end the following:

- "(6) For purposes of paragraph (r)(1)(B), a statement for a dietary supplement may be made if—
    - ○ "(A) the statement claims a benefit related to a classical nutrient deficiency disease and discloses the prevalence of such disease in the United States, describes the role of a nutrient or dietary ingredient intended to affect the structure or function in humans, characterizes the documented mechanism by which a nutrient or dietary ingredient acts to maintain such structure or function, or describes general well-being from consumption of a nutrient or dietary ingredient,

- ○ "(B) the manufacturer of the dietary supplement has substantiation that such statement is truthful and not misleading, and
- ○ "(C) the statement contains, prominently displayed and in boldface type, the following: "This statement has not been evaluated by the Food and Drug Administration. This product is not intended to diagnose, treat, cure, or prevent any disease.".

A statement under this subparagraph may not claim to diagnose, mitigate, treat, cure, or prevent a specific disease or class of diseases. If the manufacturer of a dietary supplement proposes to make a statement described in the first sentence of this subparagraph in the labeling of the dietary supplement, the manufacturer shall notify the Secretary no later than 30 days after the first marketing of the dietary supplement with such statement that such a statement is being made.".

§7. Dietary Supplement Ingredient Labeling and Nutrition Information Labeling.

- **(a) MISBRANDED SUPPLEMENTS.**—Section 403 (21 U.S.C. 343) is amended by adding at the end the following: "(s) If—
  - ○ "(1) it is a dietary supplement; and
  - ○ "(2)(A) the label or labeling of the supplement fails to list—
    - "(i) the name of each ingredient of the supplement that is described in section 201(ff); and
    - "(ii)(I) the quantity of each such ingredient; or

- - "(II) with respect to a proprietary blend of such ingredients, the total quantity of all ingredients in the blend;
  - "(B) the label or labeling of the dietary supplement fails to identify the product by using the term 'dietary supplement', which term may be modified with the name of such an ingredient;

    "(C) the supplement contains an ingredient described in section 201(ff)(1)(C), and the label or labeling of the supplement fails to identify any part of the plant from which the ingredient is derived;
  - "(D) the supplement—
    - "(i) is covered by the specifications of an official compendium;
    - "(ii) is represented as conforming to the specifications of an official compendium; and
    - "(iii) fails to so conform; or
  - "(E) the supplement—
    - "(i) is not covered by the specifications of an official compendium; and
    - "(ii)(I) fails to have the identity and strength that the supplement is represented to have; or
    - "(II) fails to meet the quality (including tablet or capsule disintegration), purity, or compositional specifications, based on validated assay or other appropriate methods, that the supplement is represented to meet.".

- **(b) Supplement Listing on Nutrition Labeling.** Section 403(q)(5)(F) (21 U.S.C. 343(q)(5)(F)) is amended to read as follows:
  - "(F) A dietary supplement product (including a food to which section 411 applies) shall comply with the requirements of subparagraphs (1) and (2) in a

manner which is appropriate for the product and which is specified in regulations of the Secretary which shall provide that—

- "(i) nutrition information shall first list those dietary ingredients that are present in the product in a significant amount and for which a recommendation for daily consumption has been established by the Secretary, except that a dietary ingredient shall not be required to be listed if it is not present in a significant amount, and shall list any other dietary ingredient present and identified as having no such recommendation;
- "(ii) the listing of dietary ingredients shall include the quantity of each such ingredient (or of a proprietary blend of such ingredients) per serving;
- "(iii) the listing of dietary ingredients may include the source of a dietary ingredient; and
- "(iv) the nutrition information shall immediately precede the ingredient information required under subclause (i), except that no ingredient identified pursuant to subclause (i) shall be required to be identified a second time.".

- (c) **Percentage Level Claims.** Section 403(r)(2) (21 U.S.C. 343(r)(2)) is amended by adding after clause (E) the following:
  - "(F) Subclause (i) clause (A) does not apply to a statement in the labeling of a dietary supplement that characterizes the percentage level of a dietary ingredient for which the Secretary has not established a reference daily intake, daily recommended value, or other recommendation for daily consumption.".

- **(d) Vitamins and Minerals.** Section 411(b)(2) (21 U.S.C. 350(b)(2)) is amended—
  - (1) by striking "vitamins or minerals" and inserting "dietary supplement ingredients described in section 201(ff)";
  - (2) by striking "(2)(A)" and inserting "(2)"; and
  - (3) by striking subparagraph (B).
- **(e) Effective Date.** Dietary supplements—
  - (1) may be labeled after the date of the enactment of this Act in accordance with the amendments made by this section, and
  - (2) shall be labeled after December 31, 1996, in accordance with such amendments.

§8. New Dietary Ingredients.

Chapter IV of the Federal Food, Drug, and Cosmetic Act is amended by adding at the end the following:

"NEW DIETARY INGREDIENTS

- "SEC. 413. (a) IN GENERAL.—A dietary supplement which contains a new dietary ingredient shall be deemed adulterated under section 402(f) unless it meets one of the following requirements:
  - "(1) The dietary supplement contains only dietary ingredients which have been present in the food supply as an article used for food in a form in which the food has not been chemically altered.
  - "(2) There is a history of use or other evidence of safety establishing that the dietary ingredient when

used under the conditions recommended or suggested in the labeling of the dietary supplement will reasonably be expected to be safe and, at least 75 days before being introduced or delivered for introduction into interstate commerce, the manufacturer or distributor of the dietary ingredient or dietary supplement provides the Secretary with information, including any citation to published articles, which is the basis on which the manufacturer or distributor has concluded that a dietary supplement containing such dietary ingredient will reasonably be expected to be safe.

The Secretary shall keep confidential any information provided under paragraph (2) for 90 days following its receipt. After the expiration of such 90 days, the Secretary shall place such information on public display, except matters in the information which are trade secrets or otherwise confidential, commercial information.

- "(b) PETITION.—Any person may file with the Secretary a petition proposing the issuance of an order prescribing the conditions under which a new dietary ingredient under its intended conditions of use will reasonably be expected to be safe. The Secretary shall make a decision on such petition within 180 days of the date the petition is filed with the Secretary. For purposes of chapter 7 of title 5, United States Code, the decision of the Secretary shall be considered final agency action.

- "(c) DEFINITION.—For purposes of this section, the term "new dietary ingredient" means a dietary ingredient that was not marketed in the United States before October 15, 1994 and does not include any dietary ingredient which was marketed in the United States before October 15, 1994.".

§9. Good Manufacturing Practices.

Section 402 (21 U.S.C. 342), as amended by section 4, is amended by adding at the end the following:

- "(g)(1) If it is a dietary supplement and it has been prepared, packed, or held under conditions that do not meet current good manufacturing practice regulations, including regulations requiring, when necessary, expiration date labeling, issued by the Secretary under subparagraph (2).
- "(2) The Secretary may by regulation prescribe good manufacturing practices for dietary supplements. Such regulations shall be modeled after current good manufacturing practice regulations for food and may not impose standards for which there is no current and generally available analytical methodology. No standard of current good manufacturing practice may be imposed unless such standard is included in a regulation promulgated after notice and opportunity for comment in accordance with chapter 5 of title 5, United States Code.".

§10. Conforming Amendments.

- (a) SECTION 201—The last sentence of section 201(g)(1) (21 U.S.C. 321(g)(1)) is amended to read as follows: "A food or dietary supplement for which a claim, subject to sections 403(r)(1)(B) and 403(r)(3) or sections 403(r)(1)(B) and 403(r)(5)(D), is made in accordance with the requirements of section 403(r) is not a drug solely because the label or the labeling contains such a claim. A food, dietary ingredient, or dietary supplement for which a truthful and not misleading statement is made in accordance with section 403(r)(6) is not a drug under clause (C) solely because the label or the labeling contains such a statement."

- **(b) SECTION 301**—Section 301 (21 U.S.C. 331) is amended by adding at the end the following: "(u) The introduction or delivery for introduction into interstate commerce of a dietary supplement that is unsafe under section 413."

- **(c) SECTION 403**—Section 403 (21 U.S.C. 343), as amended by section 7, is amended by adding after paragraph (s) the following: "A dietary supplement shall not be deemed misbranded solely because its label or labeling contains directions or conditions of use or warnings.".

§11. Withdrawal of the Regulations and Notice.

The advance notice of proposed rulemaking concerning dietary supplements published in the Federal Register of June 18, 1993 (58 FR 33690-33700) is null and void and of no force or effect insofar as it applies to dietary supplements. The Secretary of Health and Human Services shall publish a notice in the Federal Register to revoke the item declared to be null and void and of no force or effect under subsection (a).

§12. Commission on Dietary Supplement Labels.

- **(a) ESTABLISHMENT.**—There shall be established as an independent agency within the executive branch a commission to be known as the Commission on Dietary Supplement Labels (hereafter in this section referred to as the "Commission").

- **(b) MEMBERSHIP.—**
    - ○ (1) COMPOSITION.—The Commission shall be composed of 7 members who shall be appointed by the President.
    - ○ (2) EXPERTISE REQUIREMENT.—The members of the Commission shall consist of individuals with expertise and experience in dietary supplements and in the manufacture, regulation, distribution, and use of such supplements. At least three of the members of the Commission shall be qualified by scientific training and experience to evaluate the benefits to health of the use of dietary supplements and one of such three members shall have experience in pharmacognosy, medical botany, traditional herbal medicine, or other related sciences. Members and staff of the Commission shall be without bias on the issue of dietary supplements.

- **(c) FUNCTIONS OF THE COMMISSION.**—The Commission shall conduct a study on, and provide recommendations for, the regulation of label claims and statements for dietary supplements, including the use of literature in connection with the sale of dietary supplements and procedures for the evaluation of such claims. In making such recommendations, the Commission shall evaluate how best to provide truthful, scientifically valid, and not misleading information to consumers so that such consumers may make informed and appropriate health care choices for themselves and their families.

- **(d) ADMINISTRATIVE POWERS OF THE COMMISSION.—**
    - ○ (1) HEARINGS.—The Commission may hold hearings, sit and act at such times and places, take such testimony, and receive such evidence as the

Commission considers advisable to carry out the purposes of this section.

- ○ (2) INFORMATION FROM FEDERAL AGEN-CIES.—The Commission may secure directly from any Federal department or agency such information as the Commission considers necessary to carry out the provisions of this section.
- ○ (3) AUTHORIZATION OF APPROPRIATIONS.—There are authorized to be appropriated such sums as may be necessary to carry out this section.

- **(e) REPORTS AND RECOMMENDATIONS.—**
  - ○ (1) FINAL REPORT REQUIRED.—Not later than 24 months after the date of enactment of this Act, the Commission shall prepare and submit to the President and to the Congress a final report on the study required by this section.
  - ○ (2) RECOMMENDATIONS.—The report described in paragraph (1) shall contain such recommendations, including recommendations for legislation, as the Commission deems appropriate.
  - ○ (3) ACTION ON RECOMMENDATIONS.—Within 90 days of the issuance of the report under paragraph (1), the Secretary of Health and Human Services shall publish in the Federal Register a notice of any recommendation of Commission for changes in regulations of the Secretary for the regulation of dietary supplements and shall include in such notice a notice of proposed rulemaking on such changes together with an opportunity to present views on such changes. Such rulemaking shall be completed not later than 2 years after the date of the issuance of such report. If such rulemaking is not completed on or before the expiration of such 2 years, regulations of

the Secretary published in 59 FR 395-426 on January 4, 1994, shall not be in effect.

§13. Office of Dietary Supplements.

- (a) **IN GENERAL.**—Title IV of the Public Health Service Act is amended by inserting after section 485B (42 U.S.C. 287c-3) the following:

"SUBPART 4—OFFICE OF DIETARY SUPPLEMENTS SEC. 485C. DIETARY SUPPLEMENTS.

- ○ "(a) **ESTABLISHMENT.**—The Secretary shall establish an Office of Dietary Supplements within the National Institutes of Health.

- ○ "(b) **PURPOSE.**—The purposes of the Office are—
  - "(1) to explore more fully the potential role of dietary supplements as a significant part of the efforts of the United States to improve health care; and
  - "(2) to promote scientific study of the benefits of dietary supplements in maintaining health and preventing chronic disease and other health-related conditions.

- ○ "(c) **DUTIES.**—The Director of the Office of Dietary Supplements shall—
  - "(1) conduct and coordinate scientific research within the National Institutes of Health relating to dietary supplements and the extent to which the use of dietary supplements can limit

or reduce the risk of diseases such as heart disease, cancer, birth defects, osteoporosis, cataracts, or prostatism;

- "(2) collect and compile the results of scientific research relating to dietary supplements, including scientific data from foreign sources or the Office of Alternative Medicine;

- "(3) serve as the principal advisor to the Secretary and to the Assistant Secretary for Health and provide advice to the Director of the National Institutes of Health, the Director of the Centers for Disease Control and Prevention, and the Commissioner of Food and Drugs on issues relating to dietary supplements including—

    - "(A) dietary intake regulations;
    - "(B) the safety of dietary supplements;
    - "(C) claims characterizing the relationship between—
        - "(i) dietary supplements; and
        - "(ii)(I) prevention of disease or other health-related conditions; and
        - "(II) maintenance of health; and
    - "(D) scientific issues arising in connection with the labeling and composition of dietary supplements;

- "(4) compile a database of scientific research on dietary supplements and individual nutrients; and

- "(5) coordinate funding relating to dietary supplements for the National Institutes of Health.

- ○ "**(d) DEFINITION.**—As used in this section, the term "dietary supplement" has the meaning given the term in section 201(ff) of the Federal Food, Drug, and Cosmetic Act.

- ○ "**(e) AUTHORIZATION OF APPROPRIA-TIONS.**—There are authorized to be appropriated to carry out this section $5,000,000 for fiscal year 1994 and such sums as may be necessary for each subsequent fiscal year.".

- **(b) CONFORMING AMENDMENT.**—Section 401(b)(2) of the Public Health Service Act (42 U.S.C. 281(b)(2)) is amended by adding at the end the following:
  - ○ "(E) The Office of Dietary Supplements.".

Approved October 25, 1994.

Appendix C. U.S. Pharmacopeia: Verified Dietary Supplements

For updated information about verified brands and specific dietary supplements, consult the U.S. Pharmacopeia web site at http://www.usp.org/USPVerified/.

Participating Companies

Inverness Medical Innovations
http://www.invernessmedical.com/NutritionalSupplements.cfm

Leiner Health Products
http://www.leiner.com/LEN_OurProducts/Product Descriptions/index.asp

Pharmavite, LLC
http://www.naturemade.com

Schiff Nutrition
http://www.schiffvitamins.com

Tishcon Corporation
http://www.npicenter.com/Listings/ProductShowcase.aspx

Verified Dietary Supplement Brands

Berkley & Jensen
Equaline
Kirkland Signature
Nature Made
Nutri Plus
Q-Gel
Sunmark
Tru Nature
Your Life

Appendix D. Resources

Free Resources

American Dietetic Association
http://www.eatright.org

Annual Bibliographies of Significant Advances in Dietary
Supplement Research
http://ods.od.nih.gov/Research/Annual_Bibliographies.aspx

Center for Science in the Public Interest
http://www.cspinet.org

Computer Access to Research on Dietary Supplements
http://ods.od.nih.gov/Research/CARDS_Database.aspx

Computer Retrieval of Information on Scientific
Projects
http://crisp.cit.nih.gov

Consumer Healthcare Products Association
http://www.chpa-info.org/Web/index.aspx

ConsumerLab.com
http://www.consumerlab.com

Council for Responsible Nutrition
http://www.crnusa.org

Dietary Supplement Education Alliance
http://www.npicenter.com/listings/CompanyDetail
.aspx?companyId=22078

Dietary Supplement Information Bureau
http://www.supplementinfo.org

Dietary Supplement Ingredient and Labeling Databases
http://ods.od.nih.gov/Health_Information/Dietary_
Supplement_Ingredient_and_Labeling_Databases.aspx

FirstGov for Consumers
http://www.consumer.gov/food.htm

Food and Drug Administration's Center for Food Safety and
Applied Nutrition
http://www.cfsan.fda.gov/~dms/supplmnt.html
This web site provides continually updated information
on dietary supplements, including recent announcements,
an electronic newsletter, information on warnings and
safety, instructions about reporting adverse events, consumer
education, and information for the dietary supplement
industry.

Food and Drug Administration's MedWatch Program
http://www.fda.gov/medwatch
Call toll-free 1-800-FDA-1088
MedWatch is the FDA's safety information and adverse
event reporting program, which provides clinical information
about safety issues involving prescription and over-the-
counter drugs, biologics, medical and radiation-emitting
devices, and special nutritional products. Safety alerts, recalls,
withdrawals, and important labeling changes that may affect
consumers' health are disseminated via the MedWatch web
site. In addition, MedWatch allows healthcare professionals
and consumers to report serious problems that they suspect
are associated with dietary supplements, drugs, and medical
devices.

Food and Nutrition Information Center
http://www.nal.usda.gov/fnic/etext/000015.html

Institute of Medicine of the National Academies' Food and
Nutrition Board
http://www.iom.edu/board.asp?id=3788

InteliHealth: Harvard Medical School's Consumer Health
Information
http://www.intelihealth.com/IH/ihtIH/WSIHW000/
8513/8513.html

International Bibliographic Information on Dietary
Supplements
http://ods.od.nih.gov/databases/ibids.html

International Food Information Council
http://www.ific.org

Journal of the American Dietetic Association
http://www.adajournal.org

National Center on Complementary and Alternative
Medicine
http://nccam.nih.gov

National Council Against Health Fraud
http://www.ncahf.org/index.html

National Health and Nutrition Examination Survey
http://www.cdc.gov/nchs/nhanes.htm

Natural Products Association
http://naturalproductsassoc.org

Office of Dietary Supplements
http://ods.od.nih.gov/

PubMed
http://www.ncbi.nlm.nih.gov/PubMed
   PubMed is a service of the U.S. National Library of
Medicine that includes more than 16 million citations for
biomedical articles dating back to the 1950s. PubMed includes
links to full-text articles and other related resources.

QuackWatch
http://www.quackwatch.org

U.S. Pharmacopoeia
http://www.usp.org

Organizations with Paid Memberships

American Botanical Council
http://www.herbalgram.org

Herb Research Foundation
http://www.herbs.org

Natural Standard
http://www.naturalstandard.com

Publications

Books and journals

Blumenthal, Mark, ed. *The ABC Clinical Guide to Herbs*.
Austin, Texas: The American Botanical Council, 2003, 480 pp.
   For herbal dietary supplements, *The ABC Clinical Guide to
Herbs* provides patient education sheets, single-herb mono-
graphs, and extensive references including clinical trials.
Sections including pharmacological actions, dosage and

administration, contraindications, adverse effects, and drug interactions make this a useful reference for healthcare professionals.

DerMarderosian, Ara, and Jade Beutler, eds. *The Review of Natural Products*. 3rd ed. St. Louis, Missouri: Facts and Comparisons, 2000, 869 pp.

One of the most complete collections of scientific monographs on vitamin, mineral, herbal, botanical, and other dietary supplements, this book contains detailed scientific information on botany, history, chemistry, pharmacology, and toxicology.

Duyff, Roberta Larson. *American Dietetic Association Complete Food and Nutrition Guide*. 3rd ed. Hoboken, New Jersey: John Wiley & Sons, 2007.

In addition to the section on dietary supplements, this consumer guide addresses vitamins, minerals, and common dietary supplement constituents as they should be addressed—in the context of overall diet. Look for the most recent edition available.

Foster, Steven, and Varro E. Tyler. *Tyler's Honest Herbal: A Sensible Guide to the Use of Herbs and Related Remedies*. 4th ed. New York: Haworth Herbal Press, 1999, 442 pp.

This guide contains interesting background on the origins, historic and current uses, and safety concerns of herbal dietary supplements. An excellent place to start, *Tyler's Honest Herbal* is easy to read but does not contain cutting-edge scientific data. Look for the most recent edition available.

Journal of Herbal Pharmacotherapy. Binghamton, NY: Haworth Press.

A peer-reviewed quarterly journal that includes monographs, case studies, book and literature reviews, original research, editorials, and legislative updates.

Physicians Desk Reference for Nonprescription Drugs, Dietary Supplements, and Herbs: The Definitive Guide to OTC Medications. 27th ed. Montvale, New Jersey: Thomson, 2006, 406 pp.

Published annually, this comprehensive volume provides excellent coverage of dietary supplements and herbs in addition to over-the-counter medicines. Fully cross-referenced and organized by therapeutic areas, this guide is accessible to both healthcare professionals and educated consumers.

Sarubin-Fragakis, Allison. *The Health Professional's Guide to Popular Dietary Supplements.* 2nd ed. Chicago: The American Dietetic Association, 2003, 526 pp.

Written for registered dietitians, this encyclopedic reference contains an alphabetical guide to dietary supplements including in-depth, but accessible analysis of recent scientific data. Look for the most recent edition available.

Online publications

"Buyer's Guide to Herbs and Supplements"
http://www.health.harvard.edu/special_health_reports/
Buyers_Guide_to_Herbs_and_Supplements.htm

This consumer resource deftly covers issues of health and safety, product standardization, research, and issues related to buying dietary supplements.

Natural Standard desktop version
http://www.skyscape.com/estore/ProductDetail
.aspx? ProductId=1679&WT.mc_id=59423

The desktop version of the Natural Standard web site contents, including updates for one year.

"Natural Standard Herb and Supplement Handbook: The Clinical Bottom Line"
http://www.us.elsevierhealth.com/product.jsp?isbn=0323029930&dmnum=80237&repnum=70547

A concise version of the Natural Standard web site contents, this handbook contains 91 monographs on key herbal dietary supplements. Highlights include tables on potential interactions and specific health conditions.

"Natural Standard Herb and Supplement Reference: Evidence-Based Clinical Reviews"
http://www.us.elsevierhealth.com/product.jsp?isbn=0323029949&dmnum=80237&repnum=70547

A comprehensive resource containing 98 evidence-based dietary supplement monographs. Additional features include clinical trial data, statistical analysis, potential dietary supplement interaction tables, and detailed condition-specific information.

Natural Standard monthly newsletter
http://www.naturalstandard.com

A free monthly electronic newsletter that covers news, events, practices, and policies concerning dietary supplements and other aspects of alternative medicine.

Glossary

Adequate intake (AI) An FDA-recommended average daily nutrient intake level that is assumed to be adequate based on estimates of nutrient intake by healthy people; an AI is used when a recommended dietary allowance cannot be determined.

Adulteration Addition of any substance not listed on a product label, with the intent to defraud.

Adverse effects Unintended or harmful effects caused by exposure to a chemical; also known as side effects.

Antioxidant A natural or synthetic substance that prevents or delays the process of oxidation (the adding of oxygen to a molecule), which can damage cells and lead to conditions such as cardiovascular disease or cancer.

Bioavailability The degree to which a vitamin, mineral, drug, or other substance becomes available to the target tissue after consumption.

Botanical Of or pertaining to a plant.

Carcinogen Any cancer-producing substance.

Carotenoid Any of a group of fat-soluble yellow to red pigments, including carotenes and xanthophylls.

Decoction Medicinal preparation made by steeping plants, usually the more dense parts, such as the roots and/or bark, in boiling water.

Deficiency Shortage of an essential substance such as a vitamin or mineral that may lead to various syndromes (for example, vitamin C deficiency causes scurvy).

Dietary guidelines A set of recommendations regarding the amounts and types of foods and nutrients an individual and/or group should consume to promote health. *The Dietary Guidelines for Americans* (2005) provide the latest scientifically based recommendations to promote health and reduce disease.

Dietary reference intake (DRI) A set of at least four nutrient-based reference values (including estimated average requirement, recommended dietary allowance, adequate intake, and tolerable upper intake level) that expand upon and replace the former recommended dietary allowances in the United States and the recommended nutrient intakes in Canada. DRIs can be used for assessing and planning diets.

Dietary supplement According to the Dietary Supplement Health and Education Act, a product taken by mouth that contains a dietary ingredient that is intended as a supplement to the diet; the dietary ingredient may be a vitamin, mineral, herb or other botanical, amino acid, dietary substance for use by humans to supplement the diet by increasing the total dietary intake, concentrate (such as a meal replacement or energy bar), metabolite, constituent, or extract.

Dietary Supplement Health and Education Act (DSHEA) Federal law enacted in 1994 that defines a dietary supplement and a new dietary ingredient and establishes a framework to assure safety, establish good manufacturing practices, promote truthful marketing, and regulate the sale of these products (see Appendix B).

Ergogenic Increased work output, actual and potential.

Estimated average requirement (EAR) The average daily nutrient intake level estimated to meet the requirement of half the healthy individuals in a particular life stage and gender group.

Fat-soluble vitamin Any vitamin that is soluble in fats, specifically vitamins A, D, E, and K; when consumed in excess, fat-soluble vitamins pose a greater risk of toxicity than water-soluble vitamins because they are stored in the liver.

Flavonoid Any of a large group of water-soluble plant pigments.

Food and Drug Administration (FDA) U.S. Department of Health and Human Services agency responsible for ensuring the safety and effectiveness of all foods, drugs, biologics, vaccines, and medical devices.

Food Guide Pyramid A visual nutrition guide created by the U.S. Department of Agriculture to accompany the *Dietary Guidelines for Americans*; also known as the food pyramid.

Fortification Strengthening the nutritional value of a food by adding substances such as vitamins.

Free radical An unstable (because of an unpaired electron) and highly reactive atom or molecule that is believed to accelerate the progression of chronic diseases, including cancer, cardiovascular disease, and age-related macular degeneration.

Herb Part of a plant (usually that with no woody tissue, such as the leaves) used for its aromatic, savory, or medicinal properties.

Infusion A tea made by steeping herbs in hot or cold water.

Mineral An inorganic substance that is essential to the health of the body.

Nutrient Substance, food, or food component that provides some benefit.

Nutrition Labeling and Education Act Federal law enacted in 1990 that requires all packaged foods to bear a standardized label citing ingredients and serving size and that restricts the use of health claims on labels.

Phytochemical Bioactive component of a plant that may have an effect on health when consumed.

Phytoestrogens Plant substances, usually flavonoids, that act like estrogens in the body.

Randomized, controlled trial Study design in which treatments, interventions, or enrollment into different study groups are assigned randomly. If large enough, randomized, controlled trials can avoid the problems of bias and confounding by assuring that both known and unknown variables are evenly distributed between the treatment and control groups.

Recommended dietary allowance (RDA) The average daily nutrient intake level sufficient to meet the nutrient requirement of nearly all (97 to 98 percent) healthy individuals in a particular life stage and gender group.

Side effects see "Adverse effects."

Tincture Therapeutic solution created by soaking an herb in alcohol to extract the pharmacologically active components.

Tolerable upper intake level (UL) The highest average daily nutrient intake level likely to pose no risk of adverse health effects to almost all individuals in a particular life stage and gender group. As intake increases above the UL, the potential risk of adverse health effects increases.

Toxicity Excess of a substance that may lead to adverse effects (for example, vitamin A toxicity may cause bone pain); poisonous effect.

Upper limit see "Tolerable upper intake level."

Vitamin Fat- or water-soluble organic substance that is essential in small quantities to human nutrition.

Water-soluble vitamin Any vitamin that is soluble in water, specifically all vitamins except vitamins A, D, E, and K.

Index

Understanding Health and Sickness Series
Miriam Bloom, Ph.D., General Editor

Also in this series

Addiction • Alzheimer's Disease • Anemia • Asthma • Attention
Deficit Hyperactivity Disorder • Breast Cancer Genetics • Child
Sexual Abuse • Childhood Obesity • Chronic Pain • Colon Cancer •
Cosmetic Laser Surgery • Crohn Disease and Ulcerative Colitis •
Cystic Fibrosis • Dental Health • Depression • Hepatitis • Herpes •
Mental Retardation • Migraine and Other Headaches • Multiple
Sclerosis • Panic and Other Anxiety Disorders • Sickle Cell Disease •
Stuttering